Dancing
around the

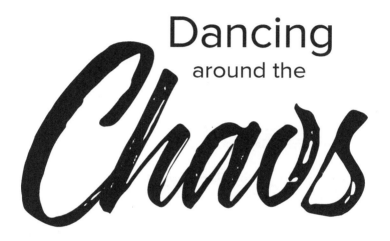

The True Story of One Couple's
Battle with Alzheimer's

TRACIE BEVERS

LUCIDBOOKS

In Loving Memory of Mom and Dad

Many waters cannot quench love;
rivers cannot sweep it away.
Song of Solomon 8:7

Table of Contents

Introduction

A man working in the grocery store stopped me just to say, "Hey, I like your shirt!" It was my purple shirt that says, "The End of Alzheimer's Starts with Me." He then shared the story of his father-in-law who had Alzheimer's, how difficult it was to watch this man he loved succumb to the disease, and how the family was growing weary. Standing in the middle of a grocery store aisle, with other shoppers maneuvering carts around us, I was reminded that this is the reason I decided years ago to write a book: people need someone to talk to so badly that they will talk to a total stranger.

Organizing a team for the Walk to End Alz was the real beginning of letting coworkers into my private, protected world of Alzheimer's. I had seen the information about the Walk on the Alzheimer's Association's website and felt motivated and excited, recognizing that although I could do nothing to change Mom's prognosis, I *could* walk. Some people feel ashamed or embarrassed to talk about Alzheimer's, while others feel they are betraying a confidence by talking about one they love and the struggle the family is facing. I was that person. At first, I was afraid that Mom wouldn't want me to talk about how we were grappling with its effect on her life. Slowly, however, I let go of this worry by remembering Mom and Dad's compassion for others, understanding they would want me to get out of my comfort zone and become that person willing to share with others just beginning their own journey. When people I didn't know well reached out to me at work, by email or over lunch, I realized that if Mom and Dad had been able, they would've listened, shared tears, and offered encouragement. I knew they would approve.

On this journey, from beginning to end, I was encouraged as friends began to share with me their own experiences. There were no life-changing answers to questions or any great news about medicine or hope for a cure; but as they shared stories of what happened with their own parents, grandparents, and spouses, I felt a strange comfort, as if I had others walking along beside me. I wasn't the first to walk this road, nor would I be the last, and I hung on to their words like a lifeline.

I found a real passion for sharing my personal experiences and what I had learned along the way, eventually inviting a representative from the Alzheimer's Association to speak to coworkers. As people took their seats, filling the room to capacity, I was taken aback: the topic no one was talking about was now open for discussion. This became an annual event, each time drawing more attendees and filling larger rooms. We were all learning that the battle didn't have to be fought alone, that there were many facing the same giant.

I am not a medical professional, but simply someone whose world changed forever when Alzheimer's disease claimed my parents. I learned from others, kept a lot of notes, captured as many memories as I could, and discovered much along the way—not just about Alzheimer's but also about real, true love. For a long time, my heart's desire has been to share my experience with others on the same journey, others who may be reaching for a lifeline.

This is my parents' story, the story of Joe and Reta.

1

Joe and Reta

I'll never forget the day Dad called to tell me about Mom's appointment with the neurologist. After the diagnosis, he said Mom looked at him with tears glistening in the corners of her eyes and simply said, "I guess this is the beginning of the end."

It had been close to fifty years since they had first met on a sunny afternoon on Reta's front porch. Joe said he knew he was in trouble when she answered the door with two-year-old me on her hip. Reta was beautiful, and it was love at first sight, the beginning of a sweet love story. Joe had two children of his own, Scarlett and Sonny, and we became a family of five when they married shortly after my third birthday.

Joe grew up as an only child on a farm near Meadow, Texas. He was raised by his grandparents and realized as a child that they had taken him in without being asked, loved him and raised him as their own, even though his parents were living. He told many stories about work and play on the farm, about racing a snake with his dog Brownie running along beside him, and about smoking his first cigarette at six years old. That farm became a part of him—the hard work of plowing fields in the spring and reaping harvests in the fall, early mornings spent in the barn milking the cow before walking to school, the strenuous but quiet job of tending the farm, loving the land. Springtime brought dust storms that picked up dirt from the plowed fields, painting the sky red, and wintertime brought snowstorms which meant shoveling snow and building fires to keep the animals warm. As a young man, he left the farm to join the Army, but he wasn't gone for long—just under a year. When Joe received notice that his grandfather had been tragically killed in a tractor accident, he was honorably discharged. With a broken heart, he headed home to take care of his grandmother and the farm, becoming the man of the house and caring for his grandmother as she had done for him. Joe had to grow up quickly, quietly picking up the pieces and carrying on, just as his grandfather had taught him.

Reta was born and raised on the Guitar Farm, about 200 miles from Joe's farm in Meadow. She had two older brothers, W.A. and Melvin, who were 13 and 11 when she was born; my grandmother told stories about the boys letting her ride on sacks of cotton while they pulled her along between rows as they worked. She loved time outdoors with her father, whether on the wheelbarrow as he pushed it through the garden or riding horses with him, checking on livestock and pasture fencing. Indoors, her mother taught her how to sew, can vegetables, fry chicken, and make homemade biscuits and peach cobbler. Reta often told the story of the day her dad came home with a radio, how they set it up on a special table and gathered around it in the evenings, leaning in to hear, marveling at this new addition to their home. The family enjoyed making music together: her parents played fiddles, and Reta, W.A., and Melvin sang along with them as Reta played the guitar. Melvin was killed in his twenties in an accident, and Reta missed him forever. He left a hole that couldn't be filled, and life for the family was different after Melvin was gone. Reta was a teenager then and dreamed of becoming a nurse and taking care of others.

When Joe and Reta got married, they raised us kids in the country, so far away from town that we were the first ones the school bus picked up in the mornings and the last ones dropped off in the evenings. We stumbled out the door in the dark after Reta filled our stomachs with a warm breakfast, and when we got home at suppertime, another good meal was waiting. We were surprised on occasion when she picked us up from school herself; this meant we were going to Ol' Jax for a Coke instead of boarding the school bus for the long ride home.

We went to a small country church, and I loved standing between Joe and Reta, listening to them sing those old gospel songs, Joe singing bass on one side and Reta singing alto on the other. Sometimes, they sang duos at the front, Joe accompanying on his guitar. A favorite was "I'll Fly Away." Their voices, like their love for each other, harmonized so that the two voices nearly blended into one.

When we were still kids, Joe got his pilot's license. Reta was afraid of flying; she trusted Joe but didn't really trust the plane. She loved being with him, though, so she climbed into the small cockpit and buckled in beside him for many afternoon flights, fingers gripping the edge of her seat, eyes tightly closed to block the views of take-off and landing.

More than flying, she enjoyed our annual summer camping trips; we all did. She and Joe donned waders and fished together in the ice-cold Pecos River, baiting hooks with smelly bait and reeling in beautiful speckled trout. We spent the evenings sitting around the campfire in lawn chairs, our feet propped on the rocks circling the fire pit, cooking fish and roasting marshmallows, while our dog barked at fireflies.

After we moved to town, our friends spent more time at our house than their own. In fact, a couple of them even called Reta "Mom." She was good at hospitality, welcomed people into our home, and cooked big meals. She always had a table full of homemade food—pot roast with carrots and potatoes; green beans cooked with onion, bacon, and sugar; fresh cantaloupe; homemade rolls; and sweet iced tea. She served all meals at the kitchen table, and supper was always ready when Joe came home from work. Sometimes after supper, he stood and offered Reta his hand, an invitation to dance, and we looked on as they two-stepped around the dog and the kitchen chairs. We loved it when we got to join, taking turns standing on Dad's feet for the dance. The dishes would have to wait until the music ended.

When I was in the sixth grade, Joe was in an oilfield accident which resulted in serious burns on his hands and face. Fire-resistant coveralls saved the rest of his body and probably his life, but he spent months in the burn center in Galveston, with Reta by his side. The first Christmas after his accident, we stacked wrapped gifts on his blankets. His burned face was coated with white cream, his hands were bandaged like boxing gloves, and he winced with pain. Even though the smell of burned skin filled the hospital room, we celebrated Christmas, thankful not only for a baby born in a manger, but for a life saved.

The days following the accident were a true hardship, filled with pain, skin grafts, rehabilitation, nightmares, and emotional strain. Reta cared for him, changing bandages, reminding him to exercise his hands, and soothing him when he woke up in the night dripping with sweat, afraid the house was burning. She was afraid, too, of what the future held, shouldering the responsibility of three teenagers and exhausted after many sleepless nights. But her love was evident to all who witnessed her tender care for him, and one day at a time, they made it through, thankful that their story didn't end with that fire. It was a turning point for them: looking back on those days often, amazed at what God had done for them.

Joe's hobby was collecting Mustangs. He was a great mechanic, learned mostly by working on old pickups and tractors on the farm; he enjoyed rebuilding old cars and getting them back on the road. Working on his Mustangs was more difficult for him after the fire, his hands tight with grafted skin and tendons that had to learn to stretch again, but it was a love that he wasn't willing to let go of. He had what we called "The Mustang Barn," which was just a place on the outskirts of town where he kept old cars and car parts and worked on them when he could. He taught others to do the same, mentoring and encouraging a love for cars. He and Reta loved going for rides together in the latest Mustang he was able to get running again. . .especially the Shelby.

The days of my youth seem like a dream now, a sweet and simple time. It was hard to imagine Joe and Reta being anything other than the mom and dad I grew up with, and really, I never tried to imagine it. After I married Troy and our kids were young, we visited them often. It was a game among our three kids to see who could spot the water tower in Big Lake first, and then the excitement kicked in: we were almost there. The kids loved going even though there wasn't much to do other than play cards or board games, walk to the park, or shop with allowance money at Dollar General. I got up early in the mornings, took my coffee to Joe and Reta's room, and sat on their bed for relaxed, early morning visits. In the evenings after supper, when the kitchen was cleaned up, we chatted on the back porch while Reta smoked her daily cigarette.

Joe still worked long, hard hours in the oilfield. He loved to tease Reta and enjoyed playing pranks on her, which even involved a snake a time or two. He was physically very strong, handsome and intelligent, and a real caregiver, quietly caring for us as he had his grandmother and many others.

Reta was a beautiful woman with a sweet heart and a great sense of humor, the very best at seeing a need and taking care of it. Many times, she fixed a plate of supper for one of us kids to walk across the street to an elderly neighbor. When babies were sick or mamas were pregnant or the elderly were ill or lonely, she was there. Joe was at the top of her list, though, and she took especially good care of him.

For 52 years, people recognized Joe and Reta as a couple who genuinely loved each other. They had good days as well as some really hard ones, but they were committed for the long haul, devoted to taking good care of each other, as well as family, neighbors, and strangers.

I would never have guessed what was coming, could not have imagined it. Had the neurologist really said Reta had Alzheimer's? A sense of dread filled my soul as the journey began. The road would be different from this point forward—nothing like we had planned.

2

Red Flags

Looking back, I remember something that should have been a red flag. Reta and I both enjoyed reading and often shared books we had read. She handed a book to me one day, but when I asked if it was a good one, she shrugged and said, "I don't really know. I couldn't focus on it; it was like I just kept reading the same page over and over again. I couldn't seem to make any progress with it so I finally gave up. I think it's supposed to be a good one though."

I was puzzled but not at all alarmed. "Do you need to get your eyes checked? Maybe you need new glasses or something." If I had been looking for Alzheimer's, I would've known to be concerned, but I had never given any thought to the possibility of this disease and knew nothing about it. Meanwhile, under the surface, plaques and tangles were quietly settling into the dark corners of Reta's mind while we went about life as usual, unaware.

Shortly after this conversation with her, Reta called Joe from the gas station, standing at the gas pump, confused because she couldn't remember how to fill up the car. They lived 75 miles from San Angelo, where most people in their small town went for shopping, doctor appointments, and eating out. Before getting on the road back home, the routine for years was to stop at the gas station on the edge of town and fill up, ensuring that no one ran out of gasoline or had to pay the much higher price per gallon at home. Reta had filled her car many times over the years, so Joe was caught off guard by her confusion. He could hear the frustration in her voice and the cold wind blowing in the background. "It's OK, hon," he said calmly. "Get back in the car and look at the dash. Can you see the gas gauge? There should be a red needle pointing either straight up or to the left or right. Do you see it? Where is it pointing?"

When she said it was pointing up, he knew she had enough gasoline to get home. "You have plenty of gas. Don't worry about filling up; just buckle up and head home. Be careful, hon. Love you." He quickly finished what he was doing in the field, headed home, and waited anxiously for her car to pull safely into the garage. After he tugged the heavy garage door down to the concrete floor, shielding them both from the cold West Texas wind, he helped her gather grocery bags, knowing trouble was looming on the horizon and that he would have to get her to the doctor soon.

Not long after this incident, we realized Reta was slowly forgetting how to cook or even how to put sandwiches together. She always, without fail, had a good meal waiting for us when we came to visit. Sometimes it was tuna sandwiches, fresh vegetables, chips, and sweet tea, and other times, it was a cooked meal—always delicious. She took great pride in preparing these meals and knew we enjoyed them. In fact, she had a reputation for taking food to people all over town for every sort of occasion, and she was always a welcome sight with fresh bread and a casserole in hand. Strangely, somewhere along the way, the meals began to change. It was odd to no longer look forward to these meals, and eventually to even hope that she had not cooked anything.

Over two summers, we had three big family events, and with each, we noticed subtle changes in her and knew we could not deny it: the decline was clearly happening. When our oldest son, Brad, got married in June 2005, Joe and Reta drove the eight hours to the wedding. I was a little worried about Joe when I found the two of them sitting outside in folding chairs, visiting with a few others after the ceremony. It was the middle of summer, hot and very humid; he used a handkerchief to mop the sweat from his forehead, and his suit felt damp when I hugged him. Only later did it occur to me that he chose to sit outside with Reta, knowing she would be more comfortable away from conversations she couldn't follow, with people she didn't recognize. Framed pictures of all of Brad and Jessica's grandparents were displayed at the reception. It had not been easy for them, but Joe and Reta had been there to witness the marriage of their grandson and his lovely bride; they had not been just framed pictures on a table.

In May of the following summer, our daughter, Deidre, graduated from high school. Our kids all graduated from a small school, each in a graduating class of around 20 students. The ceremony was more personal than in larger schools, with each graduate recognized and honored by family, friends, and teachers. After the ceremony, we celebrated Deidre by hosting a graduation party at our home, with fajitas and iced tea served outside under the trees as everyone enjoyed casual conversation. I wasn't sure they would, but Joe and Reta traveled the eight hours again to be with us. While Joe enjoyed visiting with friends that day, Reta purposely separated herself from others and didn't visit much, even with close family members she loved and hadn't seen in a long time. It was as if she were a stranger, attending a party with people she had never met before. When the party ended and everyone went home, she looked exhausted and relieved.

Later that summer, our other son, Byron, married his sweetheart, Kacie. The drive to this wedding was a little shorter for Joe and Reta since it was near Dallas, but still about four or five hours away from their home. Many friends and family traveled to the wedding, so we were surrounded by people we knew and loved. I noticed Reta seemed a little lost when it was time to be seated in the sanctuary, but our older son, Brad, calmly escorted her to her seat at the front, his hand protectively covering hers as she slipped it under his elbow. Joe followed closely behind, taking his seat beside Reta as Brad left her in his care. At the reception, Joe and Reta danced, and I watched them, remembering many dances in years past around the kitchen table. They were content, comfortable in each other's arms, smiling. They belonged together. A couple of weeks after the wedding, however, my eyes burned as I looked at a picture that captured, for the first time, a lost, blank look in my mother's eyes. Only because Joe had stayed close to her, guiding her through the evening, they were able to celebrate another beautiful marriage and to enjoy a sweet dance together, one that she likely would not remember.

Sometimes I tried to imagine what she thought at our family gatherings, where she thought she was, and even if she wondered who we were. These thoughts and worries slowly began to consume my mind, especially after I went to Reta's follow-up appointment with the neurologist.

Joe and I sat with her, waiting in the small room, feeling anxious, not knowing what would be said or how Reta would respond. When the doctor came in, he briefly introduced himself to me and then started the ugly conversation, stating very matter-of-factly, "Your mother has Alzheimer's disease. She will start declining; it will be obvious to you." He said this with no warmth or compassion in his voice, with Reta listening. I wanted to say, "This may be just a job to you, but this is my mother you're talking about!" I was still trying to wrap my head around his cold words when I heard him begin the 30-question test.

"I'm going to tell you three words. I want you to try to remember them because in a few minutes, I'm going to ask you what they were. *Apple . . . clock . . . penny.* Remember these. What day is it?"

"Thursday, I think."

"What town are we in?"

"Midland?"

"Who is the president?"

" . . . Kennedy? No, Reagan. No . . . how long ago was that? I don't think that's right. What year is it now? I don't know. Did he die?" Her brow wrinkled as she chewed on her thumbnail, and my stomach churned. President George W. Bush had begun his second term as president, and she loved the Bush family.

"How old are you?"

" . . . 70? No, 75. I'm not sure." It seemed like she needed privacy as she missed question after question, and I wished I weren't in the room. He gave her a pencil and a blank piece of paper and asked her to draw a clock. She drew a sloppy, oblong circle, with beginning and end unconnected, and then just made a few extra squiggles and lines on the page. He picked up the piece of paper and let it fall to the floor, at her feet, and asked her to pick it up, fold it in half, and hand it to him. She couldn't understand what he meant, and to her, it seemed like a rude thing for him to do—to tell her to pick up something he purposely tossed to the floor. She was irritated about the whole situation, mad tears pooling in her eyes.

"Can you tell me the three words I mentioned earlier?" he then asked.

She couldn't.

When it was finally over and we sank into the car, Reta simply said, "I hate him." I felt sick to my stomach and thought I might hate this doctor too. I dreaded what the future held and knew Joe did as well.

Over the next few weeks, we were intrigued by Joe as he talked openly, but tenderly, about Reta having Alzheimer's. One day he said, holding her hand, comforting her, "Since Mama has Alzheimer's, it's hard for her to remember sometimes. What she dreads the most is the day she will have to leave home. It'll be OK, Mama; we'll handle it. You're doing just fine."

I looked at her as she intentionally watched him talk, but there was no indication that she comprehended his words. If she understood what he was saying, she was hearing that there was a reason for this confusion and frustration, and it wasn't just her imagination. Joe was a wise man, and his choice of words was no accident. They brought comfort to her. He was becoming the real picture of the marriage vows that so many of us just recite without imagining: "for better or for worse, in sickness and in health, to love and to cherish until death do us part."

3

Communication Breakdown

Joe and Reta had a computer, but it was used only for Joe's work. Shortly before Reta's diagnosis, we convinced them that there were many other great benefits of having a computer, including email, and got them set up with an email address and a contact list. Both connected with friends and family and enjoyed sending and receiving mail, news, and pictures this way. Reta and I emailed almost daily, sharing recipes and family news. Then, at some point, I was surprised to receive an envelope in the mail from her, containing a printed email with a handwritten note at the top saying, "Wanted you to see this." I remember thinking, "I guess this isn't working that well anymore." Eventually, although email had been simple and wonderful in the beginning, it got too difficult to figure out. I realized she was avoiding the computer altogether when she was no longer reading emails I sent. Before long, old-fashioned mail in an envelope also got too hard to manage. At one point, we discovered we weren't getting what little mail she was sending because the postman couldn't read her handwriting.

Sometime after Reta was diagnosed, she asked me if I was afraid of getting Alzheimer's, and I assured her that I was not, that I had no concerns about this. I didn't want her to worry about what the future might hold for me, but I wish now that I would've been more honest with her. Maybe she was afraid and needed to talk about it, or maybe she wanted to encourage or comfort me. There are other things I wish I would have talked to her about while she was able, things I should have said to her, questions I should have asked. Sadly, I was so afraid of her realizing that we were preparing for the day when she couldn't communicate that I couldn't bring myself to do it. I wish I could ask her several questions now—names of people in old family pictures, the recipe for her Thanksgiving dressing, the thousand little things daughters ask their mothers through the years without thinking the days could end.

A few days later when I called, Reta was in tears as she told me about five Hispanic men they knew in town who had all been electrocuted.

When Joe got on the phone, he explained. "Yes, we heard news in town that a man was electrocuted when he stepped on a live wire. We didn't know him, but Mama thinks it was the five men we see often when we're making our rounds to check wells. They're always friendly to her, and she thinks the story is about them." He turned to her and said, "It's OK, Mama," and handed the phone back to her. As we were hanging up, I told her to stay warm, and she said, "I will. I have my blanket and my toothpick." I smiled, thankful for a happy ending to that sad conversation.

Every day on my drive home from work, I called Reta to chat about the day; we'd been doing this for years. I remember telling her one day that Deidre was going on a trip to the Ukraine.

"Who?"

"Deidre, your granddaughter?"

"Where is she going?"

"She's going to the Ukraine this summer with the youth group. Her friend Emily is going too."

"What? Well, OK. Mama's in the backyard picking up sticks. I guess that's fine if that's what she wants to do."

I didn't tell her when Byron got a new, exciting job offer or when Brad published a book or when I joined Troy on a business trip to London. These daily calls became too much of a struggle for her, and I eventually resorted to just asking questions that she could answer with a simple "yes" or "no."

I had read somewhere that phone conversations are just too complicated to figure out. Alz patients have a hard time understanding whom they're talking to but can't see. It was clear that this was happening. When our first grandchild was born, I didn't pick up the phone to call her, even though it was one of the happiest moments of my life. With the joy of each new grandchild came a bit of sadness. I shared with many friends and family, but not with my mother, who at one time would have treasured these calls, peppering me with questions, eager to hear every detail, her voice full of excitement. Some days when I called, Joe answered the phone and said Reta couldn't talk for one reason or another. It seemed that communication was slowly shutting down.

* * *

The Trailblazer Lunch was a regular event in Big Lake every Wednesday, and Joe and Reta never missed it. Someone in town provided the meat, and all the folks brought a dish to share and eat together in the community building. This was a time not only to enjoy a good meal together, but also to get caught up with neighbors and friends and to hear the latest news around town. Shortly after the follow-up appointment with the neurologist, I attended with them, but it was different and awkward, nothing like other times. The room smelled like brisket as everyone trickled in with their casseroles, filling the space with laughter and chatter and the sharing of recipes. Joe and Reta, however, stood around the edge of the conversation, as if an invisible fence separated them from their friends. A couple of Reta's close friends walked up and gave her a hug, asked how she was, and mentioned how great the lunch looked, and Reta smiled nervously. I watched as others waved a hello but didn't actually walk up to visit.

She had begun to withdraw from everyone except for Joe, even their longtime friends, feeling suspicious of nearly all of us. Maybe she was afraid her friends could tell she was confused, using the wrong words, getting lost in conversation, and forgetting their names. Some people did seem a little distant that day, but finally I realized they knew her well, loved her dearly, and understood that she was more comfortable without the close conversation. Joe seemed reserved and didn't talk much to others that day either. Maybe he didn't know what to say or how to answer questions, or maybe he was just getting tired. He needed to stay close to Reta, but he also really needed to be around other people. This was turning out to be a lonely journey.

4

Worry and Confusion

My trips with Troy to check on things became more frequent, and
one trip ended up being the perfect time for me to paint the house,
a long-neglected chore. When I needed something from the store,
Reta offered to go get it for me. She was still driving in their small
town at this point, and the store was only a few blocks away. She
went out the door with her purse, but when I looked out the front
window a few minutes later, she was still standing by the car, bent
over, looking in the windows. When I realized she couldn't figure
out how to open the door, I unlocked it, helped her in, and watched
her drive away. After about 20 minutes had passed, I decided to go
check on her; what should have been a very quick trip was turning
out to be much longer than necessary. It didn't take me long to find
her in the small grocery store, wandering aimlessly down aisles with
an empty basket, confused and not picking anything up. She looked
worried when her eyes met mine.

"I lost the keys to the car," she said. "I've looked everywhere,
but I can't find them! I think someone stole them."

I looked down at her grocery cart and saw the keys on top of
her purse in plain sight. I found the items we needed, put Reta in
my car, and sent a family member back to the store later to pick
hers up. She was clearly irritated with me as we drove home from
the store; it was a strange look to see in her eyes, one I seldom saw.

Shortly after this incident, Joe told her she couldn't drive anymore. She didn't like it—was angry about it, in fact.

I didn't know anyone who had parents or grandparents with Alzheimer's, or at least I had never heard anyone mention it. Maybe, on the other hand, I had just not been listening. I needed to talk to someone; I had so many questions to ask, so much to figure out. I didn't know if I should talk about Reta having Alzheimer's; it seemed like a very private matter that she might not want me discussing with others. I resorted to searching the Internet, and when I found the Alzheimer's Association, I began digging deep, finding the seven stages of the disease and figuring out where she was in the process. We were just beginning the journey and reading about the symptoms of the upcoming stages made me feel nauseated. I couldn't imagine it and didn't believe this would really happen to her.

God eventually brought to my mind Troy's uncle who had dementia. I didn't know what to say to him, how to act, or how to answer his questions that didn't make sense. One day, I was so intrigued when I saw him stop in front of a mirror and start talking, as if he were talking to a friend. He was the only person I could think of who might have also had Alzheimer's, and I had been nervous around him and tried not to talk to him. I heard no one talking about this disease in their own families, and I didn't mention it to others. When people asked about Reta, I said she was fine.

Gradually, I began connecting with others whose lives had been changed by Alzheimer's disease. A coworker told me about her grandmother with Alzheimer's who had simply disappeared. For months, the family searched frantically, called the police, checked hospitals and homeless shelters, desperate to find her, but never did. I learned that another friend at work was taking care of her aunt who had Alzheimer's, and she began to encourage me and give me regular updates on her Aunt Pat. Another friend, whose mother had deserted her as a child, was now moving her mother with Alz into her home to take care of her. Another coworker told me about a family dinner in her home, with many family members attending. She had given everyone a dog biscuit to offer their dog whenever they wanted, to keep the dog happy and friendly with so much company in the house. She looked over and noticed her Grandpa (who had Alz) eating his dog biscuit. Just as others started to notice and look at each other with raised eyebrows, she sat down beside him, took his hand, smiled, and ate hers too. Another very close friend of ours was diagnosed with frontal lobe dementia; his journey was swift and cruel.

I was finding many on this path.

* * *

Joe and Reta had long ago resorted to sleeping in separate bedrooms, thanks to Joe's snoring. When we went to see them, Reta always moved to Joe's bed so that we could sleep in hers. Deidre and I were sleeping in Reta's bed on one trip when she crawled in with us after going to the bathroom during the night. The full-size bed was much too small for three people, so I quietly got up, found a blanket and pillow in the closet, and tiptoed to the living room. Joe was snoring, alone in his bed, as I passed by his door. The couch was uncomfortable, sunken on each end where Joe and Reta sat, but firm in the middle, like there was a sawhorse underneath the couch, holding the center up high. I lay awake for hours, tossing and turning, worrying and thinking about what was happening to our family. It was plain to see that having company overnight was causing too much confusion for Reta, and I knew that would be the last time we would spend the night at the house, at least without some adjustments. Everything needed to stay consistent for her, so from that point on, we began staying at a hotel. If I went alone, I took a cot and fan with me to set up in their computer room. I spent many nights on that cot, with the fan stirring the air, in a much-too-warm house full of worry and confusion.

Reta was losing her ability to follow a conversation. She interjected comments or answers, but most of them didn't make sense or fit with what had been said. She was still wearing make-up, but it was sloppily applied—mascara on her eyelids, too much blush, no lipstick. She brushed her hair but paid no attention to the way it looked in the back, so unusual for this woman who had always been beautifully put together.

Joe was taking sweet and tender care of her but still working long hours. He loved being outside, working on his own schedule, and was good at what he did. He knew things about the West Texas oilfield that many others didn't know—the history of the wells that had been drilled out there, who drilled them, how much oil or gas they produced, and when they were shut in and why. Reta knew to stay home while he was gone but sat with eyes focused through the front glass door, toward the curb where Joe parked his truck, watching for his return. He went back to the house at noon to fix lunch for both of them. The fact that she had always fixed lunch just left her mind, and Reta quit preparing anything for him to eat. After lunch, he took a short nap with her before heading back to the field to finish checking his wells. In the evenings, they sat on the couch, her on one end and him on the other, hands joined in the middle. He often patted her hand and said, "It's going to be OK, Mama. Everything is fine, Mama."

During this time, Joe had been getting very tired and was actually not feeling well. Joe, Reta, and I loaded up in the car to go to town to see the doctor. It was spur of the moment and in the middle of flu season, so we just went to a walk-in clinic. Joe went in while I stayed in the car with Reta. She kept her eyes locked on the clinic door, asking over and over, "Where's Joe? What is Joe doing? When is Joe coming back? Where *is* Joe? Is he coming back? What is he doing?"

Eventually, I was able to move her attention away from the door, but she quickly refocused on the nearby traffic, saying every time a truck drove by, "That was Joe. Where is Joe going? What is Joe doing? Was that Joe? Did you see Joe's truck? Where is he?" She never stopped the entire time we sat there, repeating the same questions over and over, no matter how I answered. I remember thinking, "No wonder Dad is so tired."

A few weeks later, when Reta had an appointment, I took her and encouraged Joe to stay home for a bit of peace and quiet. It was an experience for me, realizing just how much guidance and direction she needed and how easily she became lost and confused. On our drive home that afternoon, she was very fidgety and kept turning to look in the back seat, wringing her hands. When I asked her what was wrong, she looked very worried and asked me, cautiously, "Where are the kids?" When my kids were little, she and I often went places with the three of them buckled into the backseat, but two were married by this time and one was in college. "Oh, they're fine. They stayed at home this time."

She looked back again and asked, with her palms turned up and shoulders shrugged, still distraught, "But where is Mamaw?"

I reached for her hand and said, "You're Mamaw; you're here with me, and everything is OK."

She visibly relaxed and turned around in her seat, settling in for the ride home. I turned my eyes back to the road, but my mind replayed her words over and over. I wanted to roll time back, with three little kids buckled into the backseat giggling over silly jokes. I wanted to enjoy fun conversation and laughter with my mother, driving down a West Texas road, with no worry about what the future was bringing to our doorstep. I missed my mom.

5

Suspicions and Doubts

When my cousin, Ann, moved to Junction several years ago and realized my grandmother's family had lived there at one time, she got interested in learning more about the family and began exploring their history. She had done many hours of research, and Reta had always loved hearing the new tidbits Ann had gleaned from her sources. Reta loved Ann, and I knew a visit to Junction could be a chance to stir up some good memories and possibly create a little joy. It was fall, and the air was crisp and cool, perfect for a short road trip. Reta was excited when I made the suggestion.

When Ann opened her front door to welcome us with hugs, I knew it would be time well spent. There was a fire in the fireplace, and the house smelled like gingerbread, stirring memories of days long ago when other family members had baked the same recipe. We sat around her antique kitchen table as Ann shared with us old pictures and family stories I had not heard before. We heard the story of my grandmother's big sister who died on her 11th birthday when she was bitten by a rattlesnake, the story of my grandparents eloping and getting married by a preacher on a dirt road, and the story about my great-great-great-grandfather who was the first sheriff of Mason County and was killed by Indians. She also told me that several years ago the two of them, Reta and Ann, had bought a headstone for one ancestor after Ann learned that she was buried in an unmarked grave, at the foot of someone else's grave. Reta had heard all of this history before, but on that day, it was all new to her. She listened carefully and clung to every word Ann shared with us, no doubt reliving her childhood, seeing her parents and grandparents in her mind, soaking up the past.

We were still sitting at the table, drinking coffee and studying old family pictures, birth certificates, and newspaper clippings, when Reta stood up and took the denim jacket that was hanging on the back of my chair, slipped her arms into the sleeves and began buttoning it up. She straightened papers on the table and carried her coffee cup to the sink. It made me nervous; there had been no indication that it was time to leave, and I wasn't sure what to do, where she thought she might be going or how I would stop her. After she was buttoned up, she headed toward the front door, waving and telling us good-bye.

When I asked her where she was going, she looked at me, slightly annoyed, as if that were a ludicrous question to ask, and said, "The bus will be here in a few minutes to take me to school. *You know that.*" It wasn't easy, but we were able to redirect her by telling her that school had been cancelled that day due to weather. I remembered that Reta's best friend in school was Hazel, and I pictured the two girls buttoning up coats and running out the door to catch the bus. Something about the smell of gingerbread, sitting at that antique table, and looking at pictures from the past took her back to a school day on the Guitar Farm.

When I was in school, I had a best friend like Hazel. Her name was Susan, and I think she ate more meals at our house than at her own. We were rarely separated; when she wasn't at my house, I was at hers. A few years ago, when Susan's mother suddenly died, she called me. It was unexpected and very sad. She had been healthy and active but died within hours after a bad fall. As I drove out to West Texas for the funeral, I thought about how awful it was that

Susan would never again be able to just pick up the phone to tell her mother something she wanted to share. As soon as the thought entered my mind, I realized that even though my mother was still living, I couldn't just pick up the phone to tell her something either. Susan and I had both lost our moms in a way.

* * *

Joe and Reta's house was starting to look dirty; it no longer had that fresh, clean smell, with beans cooking on the stove, cornbread baking in the oven, and laundry washing in the next room. When I fixed a meal, I couldn't find a fork or spoon to serve it with or a plate to put it on. We realized Reta was throwing some things away and weren't sure what was happening to the rest of it. I bought a bunch of cheap silverware and a big supply of paper goods and re-stocked the kitchen. Doing laundry was another memory that simply left her mind—it was as if a pencil eraser was slowly rubbing out memories. Joe was still working, but now he was also doing the cooking, cleaning, laundry, and grocery shopping. Home wasn't the same place anymore.

They began to eat hamburgers from Dairy Queen often. Joe told me proudly one day that he could just call DQ and say, "This is Joe," and they knew what to fix for him and had it ready to pick up at the drive-through window. When I went to see them, I always cooked a meal. One time, I took bunches of Tupperware containers and cooked most of the weekend, dividing the food into two-serving containers and proudly filling the freezer. When Byron and Kacie went to visit a couple of weeks later, Reta had pulled all of those containers out of the freezer. They were all thawed out, standing in pools of water on the countertop and dripping onto the floor.

We learned after that to take food with us each time and not try to plan too far ahead. One day, when Troy and I were making sandwiches, Reta asked what she could do to help. I wanted her to feel needed in the kitchen, the room in the house she had always loved the most, so I asked her to put some carrots on a plate. I set a plate on the countertop, with a bag of carrots next to it. She handled the carrots, ate a couple, took more carrots out of the bag, put them back in the bag, wandered around the kitchen, and put a couple on the countertop but never put any on the plate. She picked up an orange and bit into it like an apple, peeling and all. As she worked the peeling around in her mouth, she told me that her stove wasn't working.

"That thing isn't working anymore. I cooked something a few days ago, and the dish exploded! Food was all over the kitchen! What a mess—it's broken."

The stove was fairly new, so I asked her a few more questions and figured out that she had put a glass casserole dish on a burner instead of in the oven. After that, Joe unplugged the stove to be sure she didn't get hurt.

On one trip, I decided to cook a roast for supper. For as long as I could remember, Reta had cooked beans in a crockpot at least once a week, but I couldn't find it anywhere. After searching through all the cabinets, I asked her, "Mom, where is your crockpot?"

She walked into the kitchen, opened a cabinet door and pulled out a plate and asked me, "Is this a crockpot?" When I said it wasn't, she asked, "What is a crockpot?"

I described it to her, and she said she had never heard of it. All afternoon, she brought me various items from the kitchen (a bowl, a recipe box, a mixer) and asked, "Is *this* a crockpot?" My niece, Nancy, lived across the street, so I borrowed one from her. Reta studied it carefully and said she had never seen one before.

I mentioned a recipe that Reta cooked often when I was growing up, but she didn't remember it. "Are you sure, Mom? Remember? Wanda gave you that recipe for Green Enchilada Casserole. You made it all the time, and we loved it! Remember—first, you brown hamburger meat with chopped onion." But I couldn't bring the memory back, no matter how many ingredients I listed or details I filled in. It took a while for me to learn that no amount of cajoling and coaxing would make memories come back; they were simply gone.

Reta was confused and growing more suspicious of all of us. She held on to her purse all the time, afraid someone (even one of us) might steal it. To be on the safe side, she hid it, and five minutes later, when she realized she didn't have it on her lap, she thought someone had stolen it. When we found it, always in a new and different hiding place, we gave it back to her and watched her take all the contents out, one by one, to make sure nothing was missing. The contents were a spoon, an empty wallet, a toothbrush wrapped in foil, some old lotion, a pencil, a small bottle of toothpicks and a Kleenex. As soon as she had checked all the contents and tucked them safely back into her purse, she hid it again to keep anyone from stealing it. Five minutes later, she had no memory of hiding it, and the cycle started over. This happened over and over all day, every day. We could not steer her in a different direction, no matter how hard we tried.

With suspicion and confusion looming in Reta's mind, Joe was afraid to leave her alone at home and started taking her with him to check his wells. The rides were quiet as they drove over rocky dirt roads, opening and closing property gates, taking in the sights of rabbits hopping through tumbleweeds, and along the way, feeding deer from the buckets of corn kept in the back of the truck.

We went to Big Lake for Reta's birthday in January of 2011. Most of our family went with us, including our seven-month-old grandson, Max. We took a birthday cake, candles, party plates, and napkins. Reta was puzzled by the day but enjoyed it. She looked directly at Troy, confusion in her eyes, and asked him, "Where's Troy?"

He said gently and clearly, "I'm Troy, and I'm right here."

She took his word for it, chuckling, and said, "Good!"

No conversation that day made sense, and Joe was growing more weary. Reta's posture had changed: she was sort of slumped into the couch, not sitting up—this woman who all my life had reminded me to stand up straight.

After the kids left that afternoon and the kitchen was cleaned up, I asked her if she would like a little piece of cake. She walked into the kitchen with me to fix it. While I was cutting the cake, I saw her open the dishwasher and bend down to look inside. "What are you looking for, Mom?" She looked at me as if I should know and said, "A little piece of cake."

About a month later, I noticed that Reta hadn't bathed in several days. I decided to visit with her about it and then help her take a bath. "Mom, if I get the bath water ready and get a gown out for you, would you like to take a bath?" I didn't expect her quick response: "No."

"Are you sure? It's a good night for a bath, and I would be glad to help you."

She responded, "No, I don't see the point."

I pressed on. "Well, I think you would feel better if you bathed. You always taught me to bathe every day, and I don't think you've had a bath in a few days."

I wasn't prepared for the look in her eyes, "Are you saying that I *need* a bath? I don't appreciate it one bit. I'll bathe when I want to. I can do it myself." I didn't expect it to be an easy conversation but didn't anticipate her anger either. I hated the whole useless conversation about a bath that still didn't happen and went to bed that night feeling like a child who had been scolded, wishing I had never brought up baths. I learned later that this is common for people with dementia. There are too many steps to take: unzipping, unbuttoning, turning on water to the right temperature, getting a washrag and soap, getting out of the tub, getting a towel, drying off, and getting dressed again. It was just too big of a job, too many steps that she couldn't process.

The next day, I went with Joe and Reta to the doctor, and when it was time for Reta's lab work, I went back with her. The nurse said she would need a urine sample and handed Reta a cup. I asked her if she needed help. She had forgotten our bath conversation, but still answered me with a clear, short response, "No, I do not."

When she came out of the bathroom without the cup, I asked where it was. She was puzzled. "What do you mean? I didn't know about that. What cup? No one told me that." When I put the cup back in her hand, she acted like it was the first time she had seen it.

Chaos and confusion were ramping up, and I was worried about leaving them. A few nights after we were back home, Joe called and asked me to talk to Reta because she was mad and refused to go to bed. He was beyond exhausted and couldn't reason with her. I tried, but she wouldn't listen to anything I said. We never figured out the reason for the anger, but there was no doubt she was seriously mad about something. Joe and I talked that night about requesting some meds for calming her down when necessary. I wanted to get in the car that night and drive to Big Lake but, by this time, had learned there was a good chance that everything would be forgotten by morning. Evenings were the worst due to sundowning—the ramping up of confusion, agitation, and aggression late in the day, while symptoms are usually less obvious earlier in the day. I realized that my bath conversation with her a few days earlier might have gone a lot more smoothly had I attempted it in the morning, rather than the evening. I slept little that night and felt sure Joe's night was a sleepless one as well.

We needed to get help for Joe, but when we talked to him about it, he always declined, insisting things were going well. Two of his favorite sayings were, "We're in good shape for the shape we're in!" and "I'm tickled pink!" He always answered this way, but I didn't believe it anymore.

6

Fears and Laughter

If I'm honest, I must admit that I do worry some about developing Alzheimer's myself. When I forget something, just anything, I sometimes find myself looking at family or friends, thinking, "I hope they don't think I'm getting Alzheimer's." For several months, I spent a lot of time testing myself. When I walked through my office building and passed people I had worked with in previous years, I practiced pulling up names and titles from my memory banks: "Tom Belden—Production Engineer; Lindsey Jones—Manager; Jessica Morris—Geologist; Rick Williams—Landman." I tried to name every person I passed. No one knew I was doing this, of course, but it was a never-ending tickertape scrolling across my mind. When there was a moment sitting in traffic or standing in line at the bank or grocery store, I practiced counting backwards from 100 by sevens. So, even though I told people I wasn't worried about Alz, I was.

Finally, one day I realized that, by constantly testing myself, I was letting this monster wedge his toe in the door, allowing an easy entrance into my mind, even though I don't have Alzheimer's and hopefully never will. Still, sometimes I find myself searching for a distant memory of something but then remind myself that I've always been forgetful and never had a great memory for things from the past. Even when my kids were young and still at home, I would tell them stories that I had already told them. Sometimes, I know I've told the story but am just not sure who I told it to!

All my life, I've also had a terrible sense of direction and have easily gotten lost. Now, when I find myself searching for the right route, a familiar landmark, or simply a compass, it does worry me a bit until I remember that, oh yeah, I've been getting lost all my life! I don't always tell people now when I get lost, though, because I don't want anyone else to think it means anything. I do depend on my phone's GPS, as well as the navigation system in my car, but most people I know do. I'm not worried.

I've been asked several times if I had considered genetic testing. I understand that early detection could mean starting medication earlier, possibly delaying the effects of the disease, and many are proponents of testing for this reason. I've spent a lot of time thinking about it and have chosen not to do it. Each person must make this decision for him or herself, and my decision is strictly my own, not based on anything other than personal preference. I know what to do to limit my risk, and I choose to focus on that. If I were tested and told that I had the gene, I'm afraid it would affect how I live the rest of my years. I can't imagine living the remaining 20 to 30 or more years anticipating life, and death, with Alzheimer's. I think about it enough, knowing my mother had it, and see no point in adding more anxiety—for me or for my family. I've read about the need for counseling before and after testing, probably for this very reason. Perhaps it's a mistake, but for now, I choose not to do it.

* * *

It was becoming very obvious that Joe needed help, so I started making calls, searching for someone who could help take care of Reta. I talked to a Home Health Care nurse named Janice whose number I found in the Yellow Pages. She talked to me as if she had nothing more important to do and helped me understand what was going on in Reta's mind and also in Joe's, as the caregiver.

I convinced Joe that we needed Janice's help, and soon she was going to the house two to three times a week to check on Reta and bathe her. She was a lifesaver, someone I counted on for three years. Joe, thankfully, loved her too. I was impressed with how she did things; she would simply say, "Come on, Reta; let's go get some towels and get ready for a bath," and amazingly, Reta would get up and go with her. One day when Reta had her purse on her shoulder, Janice said teasingly, "Let me hold your purse," and winked at me. Reta smiled, but I could see her mind working, stirring up doubtful, suspicious thoughts. Later, when I couldn't get comfortable in my chair, I stood up to take a look at the cushion. Under it was my mother's purse. She had hidden it from Janice, and to be extra safe that day, she even hid my purse.

In May of 2011, my aunt and a cousin drove out to West Texas to visit and checked into the small motel in town. Joe needed to go to the field to check on things, so he left Reta safely in their hands. When I called that afternoon, Reta happily told me, "Some travelers came through for a visit today," as if she had no idea who they were. Strange travelers or not, she enjoyed their visit, and it was good for Joe too. He never said it, but I knew he was getting desperate for breaks like this. Caregiving is a hard job—too hard on some days.

Although caregiving took a toll on him, he was always patient with Reta. One night, after the kitchen was cleaned up, I sat in the living room with them, thankful to be near the end of a tiring day, filled with lots of strange conversation. Joe and Reta sat in their usual places on the couch, hands joined in the middle. Reta noticed a scratch on Joe's knee and asked what happened. Joe explained, "Oh, I just scraped it against the toolbox in the garage today."

About three minutes later, she looked at it again, as if she were seeing it for the first time, and asked, "Oh, what happened to your knee?"

Very patiently, Joe explained, "Oh, I just scraped it against the toolbox in the garage."

About three minutes later, she asked again, "Joe, what did you do to your knee?"

He explained again with no frustration in his voice, just sweet patience, as if he were answering her for the first time.

* * *

Reta's doctor had ordered a CT scan and mammogram, just to rule out the possibility of any hidden health issues that could be contributing to her decline. I took her to town and encouraged Joe to stay home. Considering the miles to San Angelo, I knew we would be gone three or four hours, which meant he would have a good bit of time to do whatever he needed or wanted. When we got to the clinic and I opened the car door for Reta to get out, she seemed to have no idea what we were doing, although we had just talked about it. We checked in, and the receptionist gave her instructions: "Take this gown, go to the dressing room, change, and put your clothes in the locker. Keep the key, and then go down the hall and wait to be called by the technician."

Reta took the gown and just turned and looked at me, searching for the next step in the process. I took her arm and guided her to the dressing room and pulled the curtain closed. Standing in the small, cramped space, I helped her sit down, pulled off her shoes, tugged her shirt over her head, then took her hands to help lift her to a standing position, and continued the process of undressing. Finally, after I tied her gown in the back, we stored her things in the locker and made our way to the waiting area. It seemed too warm in the room, but I knew I was likely the only one who was sweating, turning that locker key over and over in my hand with a thousand new worries running through my mind.

When it was finally her turn, I got up to follow her, but the technician directed me to sit down. "You can wait here. We can do this," she said as she gave Reta a reassuring smile and pat on her shoulder.

Reta smiled too.

Less than a minute later, the door opened again and the technician, looking not quite as self-confident, motioned for me to come in to assist her. She needed me after all.

* * *

The days weren't always bleak. One Sunday afternoon when I called and asked Reta how her day had been, her response was, "It was fine, but I thought the Dallas Cowboys never would go home!"

I laughed out loud, thinking of Reta's brain picturing that football game being played right in the living room, at the foot of their recliners, touchdowns and tackles and whistles blowing.

Gradually, I was learning that it was OK to laugh, and it felt good! I remembered that Reta had a real sense of humor and loved laughter, and I determined that I wouldn't let laughter leave her life entirely. At times, there were long stretches between laughs, so I resolved that I would jump at chances when I saw them. Mixed in with the heartbreaks, there were some funny happenings along the way, and laughter was good medicine for all of us.

One day, Reta sat on the couch, holding the dog in her lap with a baby blanket wrapped snugly around her, petting her ears. Suddenly, with hands on the dog's ears, she looked at me and asked, "Would you like to taste some of these pecans?"

I smiled, realizing the dog was actually the color of a pecan shell, and said I was too full.

Reta said, "Well, OK then," not understanding how I could possibly pass up pecans.

Later, she and I were standing in the kitchen when I brought her attention to the family pictures on the fridge. She studied them as if she were seeing them for the first time. It had been a good day for her, and I imagined family memories stirring in her mind when suddenly she pointed to a picture that we had taken of her on her birthday, sitting on the couch holding Chelsea, their Chihuahua, in one arm and seven-month-old Max, her great-grandson, in the other. She said, "I'll tell you one thing: those two are the spitting image of each other!"

I couldn't help it. I cracked up! She looked confused for a few seconds and then joined me in the laugh. When I said I was glad to see she still had her sense of humor, she said, "I like sense of humors!" and giggled some more. It felt good to laugh, especially with her. One time when I was thinking about how she didn't remember our visits after we left, Troy reminded me that even if she couldn't remember the specifics or perhaps anything at all, she had been happy for a while, and that happiness may have lingered for a bit, even if she didn't know why. Maybe this moment lingered a while for her; it did for me.

If Reta looked at pictures of Max, she later believed he had actually been there and would tell stories of what she did with him. She told me at one point, "I was sitting in the car, looking at his pictures, when all of a sudden, he just popped up! We played with the blocks, and he just laughed and laughed when they fell down. Before I put him down for a nap, I fixed him some lunch; he just loves grated cheese!" She chuckled and slapped her hand on her knee as she told these bizarre tales, thoroughly enjoying the time she believed she had spent with a baby boy.

She propped one picture of Max up beside the lamp in the living room and seemed to think he was actually sitting there beside her. She said, "I moved him once, and he didn't like it very much. If he's fussy, I just take him out in the backyard, and soon he's just jabbering away!"

I watched as she picked up his picture and opened the back screen door, taking Max out to play for a while in the backyard. I finally learned to go along with these wild conversations instead of trying to help her understand reality; this made life easier for her and for me, and I so wish I had learned this sooner. The turning point for me was when I read the book *Still Alice*.

We never went back to the neurologist but continued on with the doctor Joe and Reta had gone to for years. Joe was very protective of Reta and wanted people, even the doctor, to think that she was doing just fine. I sat, speechless, listening to Joe proudly report to the doctor, "In the past six months, the decline has only been about, oh, a half of a percent. She forgets the grandkids' names on occasion, but that's completely normal at our age."

Finally, I got the chance to interject, "What does it mean when she imagines people who aren't there?"

Joe changed the subject right away, with a bit of a frown. "Mama's doing real good; she's doing just fine."

The tests they had done a few weeks prior revealed no other physical issues, but she continued to lose weight for no apparent reason. That night back at the house, I was exhausted and ready to go to bed. When I bent over Reta, sitting on the couch, to kiss her good night, she took my hands in hers, looked in my eyes, and asked, "How's your mother doing?"

I smiled, "Mama's doing real good; she's doing just fine."

7

Puzzling Conversations

When Reta opened the door to let us in, she pressed her wedding ring into my hand, "I want you to have this. Take it home with you." She must have been watching the door, knowing she had a mission to accomplish as soon as we walked in. I didn't feel right about taking it then, wasn't even sure Joe wanted me to. But I knew that she felt like she needed to do it, that if she didn't, she might not think of it later. I knew that it could have ended up in the trash, along with all the silverware and dishes she was throwing away, so I took it and thanked her. I didn't wear it; I just put it away in a safe place, thankful to have it and understanding her sense of urgency to get it to me.

Joe told us he had lost his two rings. They didn't have a lot of expensive jewelry—the wedding ring Reta had just given to me, Joe's two gold rings, and his Rolex watch, beaten up and dirty after years spent in the oilfield. After searching high and low for hours, I finally found his rings in the garage, in the middle of dirty car parts and greasy tools, in two different places. I couldn't believe it when I found them, and Joe couldn't figure out how in the world they got there.

A couple of years before Reta's diagnosis, Joe had shared with their doctor that he was worried about his memory. He was in his late sixties and didn't think he was remembering things as he once had. She started him on a beginning dose of Aricept that day, and he had faithfully taken his medicine since. I believed his issues were likely just due to the fact that he couldn't hear well, and for some reason, it seemed like we shouldn't talk about it. He never used the word *Alzheimer's*, and he actually seemed fine.

A cousin told me not to worry about him when I mentioned that he was on Aricept. She said something about it being no big deal if you forget where your keys *are*, but it is a big deal if you forget what your keys are *for*. I knew at the time that Joe was just fine; he easily passed this "keys" test.

He loved animals, and animals loved him. Months earlier, he'd found two kittens out in the field and brought them home, the beginning of an enormous problem. When I asked Reta one day about the cats, she said, "I'm going to put you outside to spend some time with them if it isn't raining," and she literally got up and carried the phone to the backyard.

She had a hard time talking to me that day, stalling at mid-sentence several times, and handing the phone to Joe to finish her thoughts. He, of course, just had to guess at what those thoughts might have been, and she was a little frustrated that he seemed to have none of the correct words. As I hung up the phone, I found myself worried about Joe for the first time. He seemed off, and I wasn't sure if it was fatigue, stress, difficulty hearing, or just age. I thought about the medicine he had been taking, and my stomach knotted as more worry settled into my mind.

At Reta's next appointment a few weeks later, Joe continued to answer all questions as if everything were fine: "Mama is doing a good job for us, and she realizes it. Sure, she falters, now and then, but just look how far she is ahead of some of the others. She is going down so very slowly, it's hard to tell."

I was the only one volunteering any real information, and this was from my tiny window of knowledge, so I felt awkward. Reta hadn't wanted to eat for the past seven to ten days, but she seemed better now and was in a good mood. The doctor discussed plans for either full-time care at home or at the Big Lake Care Center, the local nursing home. All Joe could think about, however, was how happy he was that she was better than she had been in a week. He must not have heard or acknowledged anything the doctor said about professional care because as we walked out, he said, "I'm tickled pink!"

We gradually learned that Joe was able to really pull himself together for our short visits and make everything appear fairly normal, which worked especially well when he was actually taking his medicine. We eventually realized that he must have been totally exhausted when we left. He gave it all he had for the few hours we were there, and he did a good job of it. This caused us to go back and forth for quite a while, wondering if he really was having memory issues or if it was just his hearing. He had been calling everyone "Buddy" or "Neighbor" for years, seldom using actual names. He was very good at this.

The two cats he had brought home from the field had become eight or more cats. Joe kept saying he was going to give them away, but we continued to see cats everywhere. I convinced him finally to choose a couple of them to keep, get them fixed, and get rid of the others. He agreed, and I made arrangements for the favorite female to be spayed, relieved that we had a plan. Joe, however, didn't show up for the appointment at the vet's office; he either forgot the plan or never intended to follow through—I wasn't sure. One day he told me, "Sometimes the dog won't let the cats eat," and he smiled, wondering over this predicament with his animals. Reta said, "Hmmm, maybe the dog will eat the cats." That, I thought, would solve a lot of our problems!

When we drove up to the house in early spring, it was good to see Joe and Reta sitting on the front porch, watching for us. Joe jumped up to help Troy carry in the groceries we had picked up on the way, and I took Joe's chair by Reta. She said, "I'm so glad y'all are here! I just wish Troy and Tracie would come."

A couple of minutes later, I complimented her on her blouse, and she said, "Thank you; Tracie gave it to me. You can ask her about it next time you see her." We rocked back and forth on the porch, continuing to talk about me as if I weren't sitting there.

After lunch, I was cleaning up the kitchen and picked up a dishrag that was folded in half with a used straw lying in the middle of it. Before I got to the trash with the straw, I felt Joe's hand on my shoulder.

"Mama thinks that straw is a baby and the rag is her cradle," he said.

I stood at the counter, putting everything back in its place, carefully folding the dishrag and placing the baby safely back in the cradle, with a lump in my throat.

Joe told me a couple of other things that ramped up my concern for both of them. While he was at the bank for a short appointment, Reta walked out of the house, down the alley, up through a neighbor's yard, and fell into their shrubs. They had helped her into the house, doctored her scratches, and waited with her for Joe's return. Then he said he got up one night and found Reta wedged between the commode and the wall. She had fallen, trying to go to the bathroom. Another time, he found her in the bedroom closet, thinking it was the bathroom.

Joe took a lot of pride in caring for Reta, and changing things would make him feel like a failure. But we were afraid for their safety. Joe was losing track and needed to be reevaluated as well. We didn't believe he could continue caring for Reta much longer, but he had told Troy earlier that he equated the Care Center with giving up and had no plans to do anything other than what they were doing.

I tried to make things easier for him by paying someone in the family to check on them but wasn't sure how this was really working.

Joe was still in charge, and he let others know there was no need to come by the house. He declined the offer for Meals on Wheels, saying he didn't want to plan their days around meal deliveries. We knew he really just didn't want people in town to know he needed help; he was used to being the one giving, not receiving. We didn't know where to start but knew that something had to change before long. Each time we left them, it got a little harder, knowing there was so much distance between us.

Things were changing quickly, and time between our visits was getting shorter. Reta told me on the phone that she was cold and wet, and she seemed very confused. I couldn't get any more information from her, so I wasn't sure what was going on. When we got there, she was making no sense at all and not participating in conversation much. Joe was completely exhausted and didn't look well. When Reta staggered into the living room only half dressed, I jumped up to cover her with a quilt, turning her back toward her room to help her dress.

Janice, the Home Health Care nurse, had told me from the beginning that their goal was to bridge the gap between home and the next step, and to help the family make that step. She had told me recently, more than once, that it was time, but I didn't want to face this reality. I remembered when Joe had said Reta dreaded the day she had to leave home, and I couldn't imagine taking this dreadful step. I wasn't even sure Joe would agree to it. We had talked about getting more help for him, but he always insisted that he was fine and didn't need the help.

Things were falling apart. The monster was getting ahead, and we were losing ground quickly. I imagined a tug-of-war game with our end of the rope frayed, just thin, stringy parts of rope, slick with our sweat. We were hanging on to it with all our strength, but our hands blistered as we edged toward the line drawn in the dirt.

8

Decision Time

A friend suggested I talk to Jill, a young nurse in Big Lake, who encouraged me to seek help for Reta, which would also be helpful for Joe. She spent an hour on the phone with me, assuring me that the Care Center in town would take good care of her. Although I was a stranger she would never meet, she knew Joe and Reta and helped us turn a corner on this journey.

Long before she was sick, Reta had taken me to the Care Center and given me a tour; she was so proud of it. I went with her to visit her friends several times, and she pointed out the courtyard and the family living area, saying, "I love this place. When it's time, you just bring me here." Troy and I knew it was time.

We realized the decision was just too much for Joe. He would never do it, but it had to happen. When we went back out to Big Lake, I asked him to go for a drive with me. He was happy to go; it was good for him to get out of the house and away from caregiving for a few minutes. When we got back to the house, we sat in the car for a while and talked. I felt nervous and afraid as I told him, "Dad, we're worried about Mom. She's losing ground quickly, and we can't give her the care she needs at home anymore. We're worried about you too. The caregiving is taking a toll on you, and I couldn't bear it if we lost you."

He was listening with tears welling in his eyes. I hated hearing the words I had to say. "Dad, we're coming back next weekend to move Mom to the Care Center."

He simply said, "OK," as tears spilled down his face.

We hugged, both scared, heartsick, and exhausted.

Troy and I realized that, even with tears falling, Joe felt some relief. He had needed someone to make this decision, and he was thankful it didn't have to be him. I didn't want him to feel as if he had failed as a caregiver, because nothing could be further from the truth. He was so good with Reta, always reassuring her that everything would be OK, even when she sometimes looked at him as if she couldn't stand him. I understood that it's usually the person who is the closest, the one who gives the most care, who receives the brunt of the anger and frustration from the patient; I hoped Joe understood this too. He had been through a lot, and in fact, he had not been "in good shape for the shape we're in."

The next week, I couldn't hide my emotions at work, on the verge of tears constantly. I just couldn't imagine putting my mother in the car, taking her into the nursing home, and leaving her there. My stomach was in knots, and I dreaded the next week more than anything I had faced in my life. I called Joe to be sure he really understood what would happen the following weekend and tried to reassure him again. I thanked him for all he had done and told him how much I loved him. I asked him if I could stay with him for a few days after we moved Reta, that I thought we would need each other's company. No one told me this part of life would be so hard, and I don't think anyone told him either.

Before the week was over, a close family friend, Yolanda, called to tell me that she had been at the house and was concerned. "I saw Reta eating cat food and some of the old cut up ham and chicken that was out for the dog. I got it away from her, but I don't know how much she had eaten." She loved Reta and was worried.

While it made me sick to hear her words, it was confirmation that it really was time to move Reta. I had made arrangements with the nursing home by phone and reserved a room. They explained that she would first have to see the doctor in town for an official recommendation to be placed in the nursing home. I shopped for things for her room: a bedspread, lamp, pillows, sheets, and new pajamas. We would have to gather up some of her clothes and other things when we got to Big Lake.

When we got to town, we found that Reta was having trouble with one leg. It looked as if she was retaining water; it was swollen and hurting. While she napped in the living room, I packed up some things and took pictures down from her bedroom walls to hang in her new room. Without her knowing, we went on to the nursing home and got her room all set up, as if we were getting a dorm room ready for one of the kids. I was sick with worry by the time we got back to the house and told Reta we were going to the doctor to see about her leg, that there was a chance he would put her in the hospital for a couple of days to take care of it. I didn't know how to do this.

The doctor was more direct than I had imagined when he walked in. "So, we're looking at being admitted into the Care Center?" He wasn't really participating in this game I was playing, but thankfully none of it registered with Reta. When we left his office, we simply walked across the street to the nursing home. I nervously held Reta's hand as we walked in, but she quickly let go of me so she could give shoulder pats and hugs to the people there. She was smiling, moving from one resident to the next, delivering a warm "hello" to each.

We went to her room, and she commented on how pretty it was. I took a picture of her with my phone and showed it to her. She laughed and said her hair looked like a pot of dirt full of worms. We sat in her room and visited, as if we were sitting in her living room at home. Reta didn't know she was staying, and I imagined her trying to leave with me. I was worried and in no hurry to leave.

A nurse tapped on the door and told me the nursing home had been put on lock-down; no one could leave. Big Lake is a small town; lock-downs don't happen there. When I heard what had happened, I was stunned. Jill, the young nurse who had spent so much time with me on the phone, had lost her husband. He was a deputy, checking on a domestic disturbance call, when he was shot and killed. I had planned to meet her on this trip, to thank her, but that meeting was not to happen.

When I finally left late that night, Reta simply smiled and waved, warm and cozy, tucked in bed in her new pajamas. Outside, people in town sat on curbs under the street lights, smoking cigarettes, consoling one another, and whispering about the tragedy in their little town that day. The air was thick with emotion, warm with a gentle breeze and the smell of the oilfield. I thought about the sorrow around me, most of which had nothing to do with Alzheimer's. Many people were dealing with their own heartaches. I sat in my car for a few minutes, and when I said a prayer for Jill, I thought of my friends and family members who were praying at that very moment for me and thanked God for answered prayer. Reta was safe and content.

I parked at the curb and dreaded walking in. The house was dark when I opened the door, just one lamp turned on, close to Joe. He was on the couch, without Reta on the other end, hands joined in the middle. He missed her. It felt as if there had been a death in the family. I bent over and kissed him. "Thank you, Dad, for all you've done for Mom and for me. I love you so much." No words could come from his mouth, but his tearful eyes spoke of love and sorrow.

I walked down the hall to Reta's room, closed her door, and leaned against it until I sank to the floor. Reta wasn't there, and the house didn't feel like home anymore. Many thoughts ran through my mind, not just of the woman I left at the Care Center but also of the woman who had been both mother and friend to me all my life. When I finally crawled into her bed, exhausted, all I could think about were the blank walls where her pictures should have been hanging, the first of many empty spaces she would leave behind.

$\mathcal{G}$

Facing Reality

I remembered being worried when I first learned that Joe was taking Aricept, but we had been so focused on Reta that it had been put on the back burner. There was little time to think of anything other than Reta and her needs. Now at the house with her gone, I found myself looking at Joe as he sat quietly in the living room, and I wondered if he was OK. He hadn't been keeping up with his medicine or Reta's as he once had; that had become obvious. Maybe he was just exhausted.

In the meantime, Reta settled in, very comfortable and "at home." She sat at the table with other ladies for meals and truly enjoyed the interaction with them. They didn't seem like fellow patients at all, but more like a group of older ladies at camp. Reta couldn't join in their conversations much, but she laughed when they laughed—she could understand laughter. After taking care of business in the office one afternoon, I found her in the dining room having coffee with two ladies. When I walked up, she said, "Look at my new friends! I have never laughed so much in my life!" I realized that she had been so withdrawn and secluded that deep down she missed this contact with friends. I could not have asked for an easier transition from home to here.

The following day, while I sat at the dining room table with Reta and her friends, an old-timer in town shuffled in behind his walker. The ladies commented about how they had known him in the past. One said, "You know—he kissed me once."

Another leaned in closer and whispered, "Well, he *really* kissed me one time! It was years ago; he probably doesn't remember."

The first lady threw her head back, laughing, slapped her hand on the table, and declared, "Well, it must not have been very *memorable!*"

We all laughed until there were tears!

We visited as often as we could. I hoped that Reta was getting visits from others, but one thing was certain: Joe was visiting her twice a day faithfully, had some meals there, and even took some naps in the recliner. Every time we saw him, he thanked us. He knew Reta was safe and comfortable, and he was starting to recover from the intense years of caregiving. He felt better physically, looked rested, and now realized he had been completely worn out. Still, he missed Reta.

Soon after she was settled in, someone in town contacted Joe about doing some work, and he agreed to do it. It meant long hours and lots of time in the field, but they paid him well. He was happy, feeling proud to have this job and to be making good money. The cost of Reta's care, I'm sure, was beginning to worry him.

Reta was confused and didn't make much sense in conversations, but she was happy. After visits, she never acted as if she should leave with us, but rather like we were leaving her own home. I heard her say several times, "I just love this house!" One day when Reta and I were walking from the dining room to her room, she walked around telling the other residents goodbye.

"We're getting on the road now but will try to see you again in a week or two. Take care of yourself! I love you."

"OK, Reta, see you then," they said. "Be careful on the road!"

"You take care now; don't be a stranger!"

"Oh, we'll be careful! Bye-bye!" she said, smiling and waving to them.

Later that day, when Joe came in from the field, she wanted to see his cap. He handed it to her but told her, "I wore it to the field today, hon. It smells like the oilfield." She buried her head in it, breathed in deeply, and said it smelled good to her. When I said she must miss that smell, she pulled the cap onto her head and smiled for a picture.

In March of 2013, I was surprised to hear from Lodena, the mother of two of Joe and Reta's grandsons, and, as I learned, an RN specializing in Alzheimer's care. She and my brother had divorced many years ago; I hadn't seen her in a long time but knew Joe and Reta kept up with her and still loved her very much. She had been asked to cover for the Director of Nursing at the Care Center the following day, and at the end of her day there, she texted to tell me how it went. "I just want you to know I had a fantastic day with Reta! I went early and had coffee with Joe before heading over to the Care Center. It was so good to see him! Reta didn't know me at first, but when I told her who I was, she was so happy! She was my helper all day, holding my hand as I walked around the center. She straightened papers, folded blankets, and neatly stacked magazines. She is very loved, lovable, and her personality still shines through. I appreciate the privilege of caring for her." I felt so thankful. Who would've thought it would be Lodena that God would place there so many years later?

Over the next month, the decline picked up speed. We walked in to the Care Center and found Reta sitting in a chair watching television with other residents. She was struggling to stand up when Troy walked over and offered her a hand. With tears, I watched the backs of these two people I loved, my husband and my mother, walking away from me down the hall, Troy holding onto her left arm as she steadied herself with her right hand on the rail attached to the wall. I could see that Troy was talking to her, but she never looked at him or responded, just kept shuffling down the hall beside him, never realizing who he was.

The head nurse told me they had put Reta on some medication because she had become very aggressive and angry. When I heard that she had actually hit another resident, I felt sick about it. In her right mind, Reta would never do this, and I knew she would've been devastated if she had realized it. It was hard for me to imagine until one day, I saw this irritable side of her in the dining room. When a couple of men loudly belched and burped over dinner, she slammed her hand down on the table and gave them looks that left no doubt what she thought about their lack of manners, but no words came out of her mouth.

No wonder she was cross. She really had nothing to do except sit in a chair with her muddled thoughts, gazing out the window and waiting for the next meal. I remembered reading about memory care homes that provide baby dolls for residents, and I decided to try it. After all, Reta loved babies, and she was used to being busy, not just sitting around with nothing to do. I was nervous about giving it to her, though, afraid she would feel offended by me giving her a toy. Troy suggested that I just hold the baby until she asked about it or acted curious. This worked beautifully. It didn't take Reta long to notice the baby wrapped in a blanket in my arms as I swayed back and forth, and when she leaned closer to get a look, I asked if she would like to hold her. Once I gently placed the baby in her arms, Reta never let go, believing from the beginning that it was a real baby. This was a major turning point for her; she had a job to do now. The agitation level came down immediately because she was satisfied. I had recently heard that challenging behavior results from an unmet need. This baby met a real need and changed things for all of us.

In the year and a half she was there, we watched as Reta's decline continued, little by little. I was concerned when I first realized she was seldom walking anymore, but the staff explained to me that she was so frail and unstable, they were afraid she would fall. I wanted her to try a walker, but she couldn't understand how to use it. It seemed like it was yesterday that I had watched her easily jump into Joe's truck to go to the field with him. I remembered reading about the stages of the disease and not believing they would really happen. Reta was living the stages.

10

Red Flags Again

Joe was losing ground again. I was surprised when he said that on some days he only saw Reta once. We had a long talk about the importance of taking his medicine, which he apparently had not been doing regularly. He seemed to understand and wanted to do better. Phone conversations were becoming a real struggle. He wasn't making sense, but when we tried to talk to him about it, he insisted he was fine. He had always been the one in charge, and I knew it was hard for him to listen to our questions and concerns.

Joe told me that Deidre had left a message saying she would meet him in San Angelo. He drove there to meet her, looked for her at several different locations in town, but never found her. She was surprised when I mentioned it to her. She was living in California at the time and had not left a message. Maybe he had misunderstood something she had written in a recent letter about hoping to see him soon. We weren't sure.

One day, I was out shopping when my niece called and asked if I would like to talk to Joe. I parked my shopping cart out of the way and leaned over the handle as she put him on the phone. His voice sounded flat and confused, and it alarmed me. We didn't talk long, but I knew I needed to end it and told him goodbye. He seemed relieved that the conversation was over, but when I kept hearing a loud crackling noise on the line, I asked, "Dad, are you still there?"

He said, "Yes, I don't know how to hang this thing up."

While he muttered and fiddled with the phone, I hung up. It was over, and I hoped he thought he figured it out. Sick with worry, I left my basket where it was, groceries and all, and went home.

It was around this time that I contacted Joe's CPA to clarify what was owed on an unpaid bill I had seen. He was so glad to hear my voice and make this connection to Joe, explaining that he was way behind on filing tax returns because he couldn't get any information from him. He gave me a list of documents he needed, sorted by year; this was the beginning of my relationship with the CPA and getting Joe caught up on taxes. It was an uphill battle; nothing was organized, and finding the necessary paperwork was impossible. When I asked Joe, he had no idea what the documents were, much less where they were.

He seemed more confused, and Yolanda confirmed this. She had cleaned Joe and Reta's house for years, but she was more of a friend than anything. She was probably Reta's most faithful visitor, and she stopped by the house regularly to check on Joe as well. She called me, and I braced myself when I heard concern in her voice. She said when she knocked on Joe's door, he answered, still in his pajamas. He looked at her and said with a worried frown, "I can't remember what I'm supposed to do."

She said, "Well, Mr. Johnson, you usually shave, shower, get dressed, and go check on your wells—that sort of thing." He turned from her but, in their small house, wasn't sure where the bathroom was until she pointed him in the right direction. While he was in the shower, she looked around the house to check on things. She said the dog had been wetting on Reta's bed, and she found a pillow in Joe's room soaked in pet urine.

Joe needed a caregiver, as he had been for Reta.

Reta's physical decline was also unquestionable. By April of 2013, she was in a wheelchair. Troy and I tried to move her from a couch to a recliner one day, literally a foot apart, and it was a struggle. She thought she was moving her feet, but they were just planted, not moving at all. Her brain couldn't send those signals to her legs and feet. For a long while, she hadn't made much sense, but now there were times when it was a struggle to even make out specific words. Joe was the most familiar figure to her and the one who brought her the most joy.

Back at home, Joe wasn't keeping up with his medicine, and it was obvious. We came up with several scenarios, thanks in large part to Lodena, to help him stay on track, including a calendar, a medicine organizer with an audible reminder, and friends and family stopping by the house. It seemed that each new plan worked well for a while, and then we had to regroup and come up with a new and improved one. At one point, I figured out that every few days, Joe would just dump the past few days of missed pills into his hand and take them all at once with a big swig of water.

We were growing more concerned about him and wanted to take him to the doctor. I was never sure if he had forgotten something or if he just didn't hear me. He always put his best foot forward when talking to me, working hard to make me believe he was fine. He was still working, and I thought he was still visiting Reta daily but wasn't sure. He was still very emotional about her. I emailed the doctor ahead of time with my concerns, and this became my system for communicating details to her, without Joe knowing it.

On the day of the appointment, Troy went with him. The doctor questioned him about the job and talked about how dangerous it could be to work around pump jacks and in the oilfield in general. Joe listened to her but insisted that he never got lost and was very careful. She gave him a memory test that revealed a score of "moderate to moderately severe" compared to "mild" a year ago. When she added the Exelon patch to his medication, it was a real blow to him. He remembered when he had to start putting these patches on Reta and understood what it meant.

We wanted to believe the job was so second nature to Joe that he could still do it. He struggled with the paperwork, though, which should have been very easy for him. We wondered if he followed any directions from his boss, doubting that he could hear instructions and guessing he probably couldn't remember much of what he did hear. Maybe he wasn't even going to the right wells. Things were very busy in the oilfield though—busy enough, we guessed, that they needed to keep Joe working. We knew the job would come to an end at some point and dreaded it. He was so at home in the oilfield; leaving would surely begin a real setback for him.

Our usual visits to Big Lake were on the weekends, so I seldom saw Reta's doctor. I scheduled a call with him to get an update on how she was doing, and it was a good reality check for me. I told him that when people asked about her, I usually said it was a slow decline. He reminded me, "Remember, she walked in to the Care Center when you first brought her? In a fairly short span of time, she has lost her ability to walk, and in fact, is not actually able to make her feet move at all. Everything is done for her—dressing, bathing, bathroom, and so forth. Remember, she fed herself in the beginning, but now if someone didn't physically feed her, she wouldn't eat at all. This decline is anything but slow."

He was right. The decline was real, and it was cruel.

11

Decision Time Again

Joe had a few fender-benders, more hazy thoughts, and growing suspicions of other people, including the sheriff who lived across the street. In years past, Joe had kept a gun under the front seat of his truck, but we knew he had no business with a gun at that point. One day while Joe was taking a nap, Troy went out to the truck to get it, but it wasn't there. On that same trip, we moved other guns from the house to our car and took them home. Thankfully, there were never any incidents. I couldn't think of anything much worse.

When I was struggling with the path forward for Joe, his doctor gave me a good "talking to" about my responsibility to not only protect him but to protect others whom Joe might accidentally hurt: "I knew someone once who had no business driving, but the family couldn't bring themselves to have that conversation with him. They were afraid of how he would react if they took his keys away. Sadly, he ended up having a car accident which killed innocent people. This is *your* responsibility. He is *your* father. You have to make some decisions now for the sake of safety. He should not be driving, much less living alone."

I walked out, thinking about that family and how I would never forgive myself if something like that happened with Joe.

Shortly afterward, a couple of people in town expressed concern. The sheriff called me at work to tell me he was worried about Joe, and that he was driving without insurance or a driver's license. A few days later, a man who had known Joe and Reta for many years called me. He was very nice but said without beating around the bush, "It's decision time."

Around this same time, I had a baffling conversation with Joe on the phone but was able to piece together that he had lost his job. He had worked hard all his life and loved the West Texas oilfield. This very sad turn of events would no doubt escalate his decline.

About a week later, the sheriff called again to tell me that Joe had wandered away from the house. Someone had offered him a ride; Joe refused, eventually disappeared, and no one was able to find him. I wasn't able to reach any family members, so I called Yolanda and was on the phone with her when she spotted him walking in a pasture. I heard her say, "Hey, Mr. Johnson, what are you doing?"

Joe mumbled something about looking for a crew who was doing some work for him.

Yolanda told him, "Oh, I just saw them! I told them what to do, and they have everything under control. Let's go to Dairy Queen and get a Coke."

He got in the car with her.

Yolanda was a lifesaver.

I knew our friend was right: it *was* decision time. We went back to Big Lake, but before going to the house, we stopped at the bank and used the Durable POA to complete the documents required to add me as a signer to the accounts. Joe and Reta had been so wise to set this up over 20 years before. Joe would have to sign this document; I wasn't sure how that conversation would go but had no doubt it had to happen. We hadn't told him we were coming, so he was surprised to see us. He didn't look good, wasn't clean or shaved, and his clothes were dirty—not like him at all. He was losing weight, and he had a look of panic in his eyes.

I sat beside him on the couch and asked if I could help him go through his mail; there were unpaid bills and notices from collection agencies stacked up on the coffee table, the bar, and the floor, among the piles of newspapers and other unopened mail. I started opening envelopes, and he tried to participate by shuffling papers. When we got to the bottom of the first stack, I pulled out the bank document. "Dad, this is some paperwork from the bank that I need you to sign. It will give me permission to help you pay your bills and that sort of thing."

He looked from my eyes to the paper on his lap. It was clear that he wasn't sure what I was talking about, but he trusted me. I gave him a pen and pointed to where he needed to sign. With his signature came my new responsibility for managing his banking, paying bills, and so forth.

I went right back to opening mail and sorting through bills and trash while Troy pulled up a chair in front of Joe, leaned forward, and put his hands on Joe's legs, just above his knees. His touch got Joe's attention, and Troy said, "Joe, we're concerned about your driving. Tracie and I would feel better if you didn't. We don't want you to get hurt and know you wouldn't want to hurt anyone else."

Joe responded with no sign of anxiety or frustration. "Well, I don't drive much," he said, "just around town, so it's no big deal."

Troy didn't tell him to stop driving or to hand over his keys, but gently put the ball in Joe's court. It was hard to imagine making progress with this situation, but we had at least opened the topic for more discussion later. "We'd really like to help take care of you and Reta, Joe," Troy continued. "We could move you close to us and really help with things—make it a lot easier for you."

Joe listened, but his response was clear: "No, this is our home. This is where we'll stay. Thank you, Troy."

As Joe and I continued opening mail, Troy walked across the street to the sheriff's house to update him on what was happening and to ask him to keep an extra close eye on things. He had only been out the front door for a couple of minutes when Joe reached in his pocket, pulled out his truck key, and handed it to me. He said, "Tell Troy that's the only key." I simply thanked him, put it in my pocket, and got back to the mail, not wanting to make a big deal about it. Apparently, deep down, he knew it was time, had a moment of clarity, and did what he knew he had to do. It was extra hard to leave him when it was time to go home, but we knew we would be back soon.

We quit calling because we could tell it was a struggle for him to talk on the phone. I remembered reaching this point with Reta. Family members started giving him his medicine, preparing meals, and staying with him around the clock.

One time when Scarlett, my sister, was in the yard with him and heading back into the house, he refused to go in. "I will *not* go in that house. I want to go home. Where is my house?" He felt his pockets, looking for his truck key, and pulled out a pocket knife instead. He stood in the dark at his truck for over an hour, refusing to go into the house, working to wedge the blade of his pocket knife into the keyhole of the truck door.

He was losing weight; his clothes were just hanging on him. We actually started wondering if he might have cancer or something; his physical appearance was changing so rapidly.

Joe loved animals, always had. His Chihuahua received better care than a lot of people, and she even slept in his bed. He got up earlier than she did every morning, but went back to pick her up and carry her to the living room when she barked for him to come. He fed her by hand (never dog food), and she growled at anyone who got close to Joe, fiercely baring her few remaining spindly teeth. The dog was one of my biggest worries about moving Joe to a nursing home because I knew it would break his heart to leave her behind.

Besides the dog, there were the cats. Yolanda called me to deliver the latest cat news: "Mr. Johnson set up a bed for the cats in his bathtub, and there's a new litter of kittens in there. I noticed one of the kittens was dead so I mentioned it to him. He told me you wanted it to stay in the bathtub and to leave it right there. I went ahead and took it outside, but I think he's pretty mad at me."

There would be at least two more litters born, each time getting messier and smellier. Joe was not only letting cats sleep in his bed, he was putting food in his bed for them. The nauseating smell in the house was a stark reminder of how much things had deteriorated. None of the animals was house trained, and the carpet was ruined. Joe called the cats "the kids," and I had just about had it with them. I couldn't stand seeing Joe live in such filth, and he knew I hated the cats. Not to mention, it was pretty unnerving to sit in his living room with cats running and jumping everywhere, flying through the air, chasing each other from chair to couch to coffee table.

Joe was not driving, of course, since we had the truck key. Someone told us that he was walking all over town and was no longer seeing Reta every day. He walked to Dairy Queen for hamburgers, and those were all he ate. One time when we walked into the house, we found whole hamburgers, as well as pieces of hamburgers and fries, scattered about on the floor of the house, everywhere, for the animals. Where there had been a bowl of water for them previously, there now was a bowl of Coke. When I checked the fridge, I found about 20 partly eaten hamburgers, rewrapped in DQ paper.

When Joe told Troy that the nursing home was free now, we realized that he hadn't paid them in two to three months. That was a big bill to pay, but they were understanding. "Oh, we weren't worried about it," they said. "We weren't going to bother Joe because we knew you would take care of it eventually. How's he doing? We've missed him." Small towns are amazing and refreshing. We left wondering just how long it had been since he had seen Reta.

From there, we went to the courthouse to see the judge about an outstanding traffic ticket Joe had. She expressed her concern for him, saying she drove by his house every morning just to be sure nothing looked off and offered him a ride any time she saw him walking around town. The people in Big Lake had been watching over Joe, even when we didn't understand just how great the need was.

As we made our way through town, taking care of unpaid bills and unfinished business, we learned some things we didn't know about Joe and Reta. One person in town told me that her father-in-law had died unexpectedly a few years ago, and that Joe had gone to their house to let them know he was starting a fund at the bank to pay for the funeral. Another man told us that when he was out of work and at his lowest point, Joe started picking him up every morning to ride to the field until he had him working again. When I went to the post office to see if any leftover mail was there, I ran into a young woman who hugged me when she realized who I was, saying Reta had been a friend to her at a time when she was desperate for someone to care about her. It seemed that everywhere we went, we heard another account of what Joe and Reta had done for one person or another.

When we got back to the house, I wanted to go see Reta and really wanted Joe to go since he hadn't been in a while. Sitting on the couch, I asked him how Reta was doing.

His brow wrinkled, he said, "I haven't seen her in a long time. Have you? I heard that she got a job in another town."

He looked so bewildered. I said, "Dad, Mom is here in town. She has Alzheimer's and is in the nursing home."

His mouth fell open in disbelief, and tears pooled in his eyes. "No one told me that. I didn't know. She's *here* in *this* town?"

When I said, "Let's go see her, Dad," he jumped up from the couch to go with me. As we walked down the sidewalk toward the car, he began to slow down, and I could tell he was worried.

He stopped and looked at me. "But where are we going? Tokyo?" I felt nauseated. "Dad, we are just going a few blocks from here, to the nursing home. That's where Mom is—just a short distance from the house."

When we drove up to the nursing home, the look on his face told me that he thought he was seeing it for the first time. We walked in and found Reta sitting in the living area, watching TV with other residents. Joe sat down beside her but looked lost as he searched for words to say to her, looking as if deep down, he wondered if this was really her. He wasn't making sense, but I watched Reta look at him with a slight smile on her face and knew she had missed him. It was clear that we couldn't leave him by himself any longer.

It was near the end of 2013, and the Home Health Care nurse, Janice, told me that Joe's decline was the quickest and worst she had ever seen. Scarlett told me she had gone by to check on him a couple of nights before and was surprised to see all of his clothes folded and stacked in the living room on the couch, along with other household items. He explained to her, "A truck will be picking me up tonight with the furniture and all my clothes. I'm going back home to Texas."

We made an appointment to see the doctor and were getting into the car when Joe said he would be right back and disappeared into the house. It was cold as we waited in the car, the heater running, watching the front door through foggy car windows. He finally stumbled out of the house and down the sidewalk, clutching a framed picture. He opened the car door and slid into place, saying, "Dad wants to ride with us." He carefully propped the picture of his father in the seat next to him.

The clinic was just a few blocks away. Within minutes, we were listening to the doctor tell us, "You have every reason to be concerned. He needs to get into the Care Center ASAP." His score on the mental status exam that day was 8 out of 30. There were no openings at the Care Center, but we put his name on the waiting list. Waiting for an opening was essentially waiting for someone to die. It was hard to quietly hope for an opening, knowing we didn't want someone to die, but also knowing we were growing desperate.

12

Memories in Mayhem

We couldn't wait any longer. It had been two weeks since the doctor told us that it wasn't safe for Joe to be at home. Even though it had been many years since I was a child, I realized I still wanted his permission for each step. We would have to move forward without it.

We made arrangements to take him to a nursing home in San Angelo until a room opened up in Big Lake. Troy helped him get dressed, and while I worked on getting his things together, Troy took him for a drive around town. They drove by the shop where Joe and Reta had their Hot Oil Service business for many years. When Troy asked Joe if it looked familiar to him, he shook his head and said it didn't, but as they were driving away, Joe said, "I only remember 506." This was a puzzle to Troy until he figured out that 506 was the address of the building. So interesting: Joe had always loved numbers, and the numbers were what stuck with him. He had no idea when we left the house that day that he would never go back home.

We went out to eat Mexican food and then to Baskin-Robbins for ice cream before heading over to the nursing home. Joe didn't know what we were doing, but he enjoyed the outing. He and Troy sat in the living area of the nursing home, watching TV with other residents, and Joe was friendly with everyone there. I had been in the office for about an hour working on the paperwork when I happened to see Joe go by the office door with a nurse. He caught a glimpse of me and stopped in his tracks, surprised and happy to see me, as if he hadn't seen me in weeks. He smiled, telling the nurse, "That's my sister!"

When he was finally registered, we left. It was suppertime so he was distracted with finding a chair in the dining room and settling in for a good supper with other folks. It wasn't the perfect place, but it was all we could find. We knew he would be safe, and that this would work for a couple of weeks while we waited for an opening in Big Lake.

We drove the 75 miles back to Big Lake and had been there less than half an hour when my phone rang. It was the man I had talked to at the nursing home, the one who helped with registration. He said, "Tracie, I'm calling to tell you that Joe Johnson is missing."

I couldn't believe what I was hearing; they had put a bracelet on Joe that would sound an alarm if he tried to get out. How could this happen? He was very apologetic and explained that they and the police were looking for him. It was dark and cold, and he had no coat. We headed back to San Angelo, not wanting to think about what might happen that night and praying that God would protect him. About the time we got to town, my phone rang again.

"Tracie, we found Joe, and he's here. We found him a couple of miles away, and he fought the officer who picked him up. It was a struggle to get him in the car, but he's here and OK."

Of course he put up a fight, I thought; he probably thought that he was being abducted by a stranger. I didn't understand how this happened and wanted to know the details about Joe's bracelet that should have set the alarm off.

The man on the phone apologized again. "The alarm did go off. There were a lot of visitors here at that time, and we assumed it was a family member of someone else who had set it off. This happens if someone opens the door without entering the code. I'm very sorry it happened, and we will make every effort to correct this. But, it is clear that we cannot keep Joe here. I need your verbal permission to move him tonight to a more secure, locked down facility. I'm not sure they will be able to accept him, but it is next door to us." I pictured Joe surrounded by strangers in a place he didn't know, wondering how he got there, being shuffled to yet another strange place. Worry and a sense of dread filled our car as we drove to the hotel, knowing there would be little sleep that night.

The Director of Nursing at the secure facility called a couple of hours later to tell me they had Joe safely there. "He's just fine. We're getting him set up in a room now. I have to tell you, when I went to get him, I was surprised. He looks so young and healthy—not at all what I was expecting. We'll take good care of him. Don't worry." I liked her, trusted her immediately, and was thankful Joe wasn't in the other place anymore.

The next morning, we went to the new facility to talk to the nurse at a time when Joe wouldn't see us. I started crying as she showed us around, and she hugged me as I explained that I just didn't feel like Joe belonged there. Did he? Was he like the other people I saw? I called every night to check on him, and the staff seemed to genuinely care about him. After he had been there a couple of weeks, I told a nurse on the phone that I kept thinking that maybe he was just fine, that we shouldn't have left him there.

He encouraged me. "It's natural for you to feel that way," he said. "Many families go through that same thing. Don't worry about him. He's doing fine, and we're taking good care of him. He's safe and seems to like it here." A couple of nights later when I called, the nurse said Joe happened to be sitting right there and put him on the phone. His voice sounded so strong and normal when he said "Hello?" that I was excited.

"Hey, Dad! It's me, Tracie!"

He said, "I'm sorry, hon; I don't know who you are," and handed the phone back to the nurse.

Early in January 2014, we went to check on both Joe and Reta in their separate homes. When we walked into the dining room of Reta's Care Center, we saw her across the room, strapped into a geri chair, unresponsive, with someone trying to feed her. Reality was setting in: I was losing her. My tears wouldn't stop. She didn't try to talk, and if she did, it was brief, and we couldn't understand her. Overall, we had a hard time connecting with her and left that day believing it could be our last time to see her.

We went from there to Joe's nursing home, 75 miles away. There was still no opening in Big Lake, and Joe had been there over a month. The staff was sweet and attentive, but when we visited, everyone was just sitting in chairs lined up against the wall in a hallway, outside of the dining room. I found myself wondering if this is what they did all day, moving from the hall to the dining room for meals and then back to the hall until the next meal. Joe seemed happy, talking about farming, the oilfield seemingly erased from his mind. He was sitting by a lady named Ruby whom he appeared to believe was Reta. He called her "Mama" and kept his hand on her hand, as he had always done with Reta. Ruby introduced herself to us over and over again. She was very sweet and seemed comfortable, knowing she was loved and well cared for by a nice man who may or may not have been her husband; she probably didn't know for sure. Joe would not knowingly betray Reta, this I knew, but it seemed like we were deceiving Reta and Joe both by not correcting it. Then, on the other hand, who would remember the correction an hour from now? When we left, Joe was curious about how we knew the code to the door, but he didn't try to follow us. He smiled and waved goodbye to us through the small square window in the door.

When we got into the car to go home that day, Troy reached for my hand, wet with soggy tissues and tears. "Trace, it's time to bring them home with us. I know Joe said he wanted to stay in Big Lake, but this isn't working. I don't like having them separated; you know they would not want that. We have honored his wishes, but we've stretched this out as long as we can. He trusted us to take care of them, and I don't feel like we are at this point."

He was right, and his words brought me relief. We didn't know when or how we would make this happen, but this was the road we would go down. We knew this course of action would honor their wishes.

13

Together Again

My close friend Therese told me about Delano House, where her Dad was living at the time. It was a privately owned home, and there were several of them in the Houston area, one just 10 minutes from our house. She recommended it without reservation, so I called the facility that night, thinking it would be the beginning of a long process of gathering information and then, if it was a good fit, waiting a long time for two openings. My conversation that night was close to an hour as the person at Delano House told me stories of other residents and how the staff loved them like family. She asked me about Joe and Reta and answered every question I could think of. At the end of our conversation, I made an appointment for a tour the next morning. I was surprised to hear they had two openings and wanted to be sure I was there early before one of the vacancies was filled by other families who surely were also searching.

I felt at home as soon as I walked in. A cake was baking in the oven, giving it the feel of a nice, warm, and comfortable home for 16 people, nothing like a nursing home. Some residents were watching TV while others played Bingo. One caregiver was treating a resident to a manicure, while another stood behind a wheelchair, with a curling iron and hairspray, fixing hair. I watched as one caregiver helped a lady up from her chair, saying, "Mama, it looks like you spilled your water in your lap. . .let's go change." A couple of the residents were napping in recliners, snugly wrapped in warm blankets. None of the residents was in pajamas, but all were dressed, clean, and well-groomed. It was a place overflowing with love and dignity for the folks who were spending their last days there, whether it was a month or many years. Residents and staff alike seemed content and happy. I paid the fee to reserve the two rooms for Joe and Reta and walked out, finally feeling a burden lifted as I imagined them back together in this place I loved already.

We made arrangements to have Reta moved by ambulance. I waited at Delano House, anxious for her arrival. I watched as residents finished supper, disappeared to bathe and change into bedclothes, and then returned to find a seat to watch "Wheel of Fortune." It was late, well after the television had been turned off and most residents had gone to bed, when the paramedics finally walked in carrying Reta on a stretcher. She was trying to sit up and was leaning so far to one side that it looked as if she would topple off the stretcher and onto the floor. The paramedics said she rode like this the entire way, holding onto her baby doll, looking out the window. The caregivers greeted her as if they'd been waiting for weeks for her arrival:

"Reta! We have been waiting and waiting for you!"

"We thought you would never get here!"

"Reta, is this your baby? She's so cute!"

"We are so happy you're finally here!"

Reta looked at them with a little smile, trying to figure this out. She must have been thinking, "I don't think I know these people, but I like them!"

Even though it was late, one of the caregivers took her down the hall for a bath, knowing it had been a long, hard day and that a bath would help her relax. I loved this place and went home, grateful beyond measure. Sinking into my bed, I slept deeply, better than I had in weeks.

A couple of days later, our sons, Brad and Byron, and I drove to West Texas to get Joe. The nursing home knew we were coming, and they had him ready to go, bright and early. I wanted to get him to the truck before he saw Ruby and insisted on bringing her. I had no idea what to expect, unsure if he would fight us about going toward Houston, so I asked for a sleeping pill to take with us. When Joe walked out of his room, all dressed, and saw us standing there, his face lit up. We told him we had come to take him for a ride in the truck, and the look in his eyes said it all: this was good news to him! We quickly gathered up his things without him knowing, checked him out, and headed toward the door. He couldn't believe it when we input the secret code and opened it.

"How did you do that? I couldn't figure it out," he said while looking over his shoulder, ushering us through the door before someone saw us breaking a rule and stopped us from our truck ride. He looked like a teenager, happy to be disobeying but nervous about it too.

I said, "Dad! We're busting you out!"

He laughed.

He eagerly jumped into the truck when I opened the door. To be on the safe side, we put him in the back seat so we could use the child safety locks. Joe sat up straight watching all the sights, holding my hand, and talking nonstop the entire way, snacking on Nutter Butter cookies and M&M's. He pointed out places he had seen, buildings he had painted, tractors he had driven, and wells he had drilled—even though we were a long way from his home. At one point, he told Byron, "Son, turn left at that light coming up. We'll go about two more miles before we get to I-20; then we'll head north. I'll show you when we get to that road." Byron simply responded, "Yes, sir. Thanks, Papaw," and kept driving toward Houston. It was a great drive. Joe thoroughly enjoyed all eight hours of it, and I never had to take the sleeping pill out of my pocket.

We didn't tell Joe where we were as we parked at Delano House; we all just started unbuckling and opening truck doors. I was loosening Joe's seatbelt when Troy walked up to meet us, and Joe was happy to get a warm bear hug from this man he trusted. I wondered if he thought he was at our home, but we didn't mention where we were, just started toward the door of Delano House. I was very excited for Joe to finally see Reta. She was just a few feet from the door when we walked in, in her wheelchair facing the door, obviously set up there by caregivers looking forward to the reunion. I was caught off guard as Joe looked at her and then walked past her, greeting other people, shaking hands and introducing himself. It was obvious that nothing about Reta registered with him. He didn't know her, but thankfully Reta seemed unaware of the whole situation. We slowly guided him back to her. Finally about 20 minutes later, he looked at her, eyes narrowed, as his brain finally allowed him to recognize his bride, and he broke down. The tears streamed from his eyes as he said over and over, "I forgot her. I can't believe I forgot her. I forgot Reta."

Reta smiled and reached for him. She wanted to touch him and couldn't take her eyes off him. It was very sweet, and every face in the room was wet with tears. They were safe and would be well cared for, and most importantly, they were together again, just a couple of days before their 50th wedding anniversary. So much had happened over those 50 years, good times as well as some really hard ones, but they were weathering this storm together.

As soon as Joe saw me walk in the next day, he walked up to me, put his hands firmly on my arms, looked directly into my eyes, and said, "Hon, all the doors here are locked. I haven't been able to get any of them open. I'm not sure what's going on around here, but I need to get to work. I think I'm going to have to cut the power to the place."

I responded calmly, "Dad, that sounds like a great plan. Let's talk about it after I meet with the nurse. I'll be right back. Wait for me, and I'll help you." While I was visiting with the nurse, I watched Joe through a window, checking the gate in the backyard, looking for loose boards in the fence, checking for an escape route. At the other home, they had talked about "exit-seeking behavior." I assumed this is what they meant, and it worried me. I left when I could, without him seeing me go, and we waited a few days before going back.

Twyla, the manager of Delano House, called me after a few days. "You need to come. Papaw has settled in and is doing well. It will be fine." I loved hearing her call him by his grandparent name, "Papaw." He was going to feel at home here, surrounded by people who cared for him as they would their own grandfather.

I asked if I could talk to him on the phone, and he seemed surprised to hear my voice, as if he hadn't heard from me in weeks. He didn't seem to be trying to leave. He told me, "Mama and I are just a few miles from town, and that's really good. Everything is top T, and I'm tickled pink! My wife is here with me, and they brought in some wood to fix up the place some, so I'm pretty busy. I did tell them I'm not really that good at working wood." Apparently, the maintenance man was working on some projects that day. "We love the place and are so proud of what we have." I told him I would come see him in a day or two, and he said, "My little girl, well, Tracie, has been here some." He had forgotten the drive, and I decided to go the next day; it felt safe.

The caregivers had set two recliners together for Joe and Reta in their own little cozy corner of the living room. They told me that Joe was taking care of her and didn't leave her side, explaining that he and Reta were traveling the roads and had just stopped in there for a few days. He was feeding her all of her meals, sitting next to her, holding her hand, and saying, "It's OK, Mama; everything's going to be just fine." He helped them get her ready for bed, gave them a lot of advice about how best to care for her, and stayed with her, holding her hand, until she went to sleep. He started nights out beside Reta on her twin-sized bed, barely hanging on to the edge, long legs dangling off, before moving to her fall mat on the floor. A few times, the caregivers sent me pictures of him sleeping on the loveseat in her room, his frame much too long for a loveseat but comfortable, just the same. Everyone there was intrigued by this sweet love affair, two people who had been married for 50 years, forced apart by illness, but together again.

* * *

I often fed Reta while I visited with Joe. She was alert but not making much sense. Still, it was so good to see her awake and sitting at the table for meals. What a difference from a few weeks ago.

Joe was rambling. "Something isn't right. I've lost seven or eight days." He pointed to his throat, shaking his head with a grimace. "Something isn't right."

I asked him if his throat was sore.

He said, "No, it isn't. I can't sing. I tried, and it sounded—it sounded like—spraying—squirrels." He was puzzled and worried about this, frowning. He brought it up a few times, quite seriously. I was surprised; he seemed more confused and really off. On my way out, I mentioned our conversation to Twyla, and she said they had heard him singing in the bathroom earlier.

She also told me that the day before, they had done some work in the backyard, cleaning up the patio, moving the furniture around, and so forth. Joe had gone out and helped them. Any time one of the women started to move a chair or something, he stepped in and insisted on taking over. When the work was done, they said Joe reached into his pocket, searching for truck keys, and said, "Well, it's time for me to hit the road. I'll see y'all tomorrow," as if the day's work was done and he was heading home.

They simply said, "Oh, well, the roads are icy. You better stay here tonight."

He said, "OK, but where will I sleep?"

They guided him in to his room, and he wasn't sure if he had seen it before.

One day, Brad and Jessica brought our grandsons to Delano House for a visit. It was strange watching Joe play with a beach ball with the other residents, his outstretched fingers tapping it to the next person. The boys, however, saw nothing strange—just a fun game going on in the living room—and joined in. When I looked out the window later and saw Joe carrying three-year-old Tom around the backyard, I realized how much things had changed since our move from West Texas. It had been the right thing to do.

A couple of weeks later when we walked into Delano House, Joe and Reta were in their recliners beside each other, a floor lamp between them warming the view. Joe was sound asleep, and Reta was relaxing with one foot propped up on the arm of his recliner. She was awake but not very perky, didn't seem to know us, and wasn't responding much. We talked to her for a while until Joe woke up, and then she warmed up to us. This had become the norm; she always responded to hearing Joe's voice. When we showed her a picture of our grandsons, she took her hands out from under the blanket on her lap, held the picture with both hands, and really studied it. I wondered what she thought as she looked at a picture of three baby boys, strangers to her, yet her great-grandchildren.

I said something to Joe about when we lived in the yellow house, but he didn't know what I was talking about. This was the house I grew up in back in Midland; it had also been the home of the elder President George Bush and First Lady Barbara Bush while they were raising their young family. Many years ago, Reta had written a letter to Barbara Bush about the house and was so proud of the response she received from the First Lady. We all loved the Bush family, but Joe didn't seem to know who they were that day. I showed him a picture of the house; he studied it but quickly moved on to other pictures, including the picture of him and Reta dancing at Byron's wedding. He liked the picture but didn't know who the people were. Then he said, "If I fall down and can't get up, I've had a good life." I knew he was happy whether or not he knew the people and houses in the pictures.

Joe's money was hard-earned, and he had spent a lot taking care of other people in his lifetime. He had put a good amount aside, but we needed to figure out how long it would last. We made plans to sell the house. It would require a lot of cleaning up, but thankfully the oil business was booming and several people had asked when the house would be on the market. We would also need to sell vehicles, including the Shelby, which had been his pride and joy for over thirty years. Joe had told Troy he wanted him to have it; he also told one of our sons the same thing, and we weren't sure who else he might have said this to. Nothing was written down, and the fact was that we needed the money for their care more than anyone needed the car, heartstrings or not. As hard as it was sorting through dusty boxes of personal papers, pictures, tools, clothes, keepsakes, and every manner of household item—things that had been important to them for fifty years—it had to be done. Another door to our family's past would soon close.

I didn't want Joe and Reta to go more than a couple of days without seeing a familiar face, so while we were out of town working on the house, Byron and Kacie went by to check on them. Reta was already in bed when they got there, and when they asked Joe how she was, he said, "I don't know. I'm here by myself, just for a couple of days for a job. I don't know where Mama is. I'm not actually staying here. I'm staying in an old box down the street."

When our work was finished and we got back to Delano House, we met a newly hired caregiver. She told me the story of going into the office to apply for the job and seeing Joe sitting on the office loveseat, visiting with Twyla. When he saw her, she said, "He jumped up on his feet as if he had just seen a long-lost friend, with arms wide open, and said, 'Hey, guy!' That was one of the best hugs I've ever gotten!"

Joe actually loved hanging out in the office, and there were times I think he believed he was the boss. Twyla sent me a picture once of him sitting in her place with his feet propped up on her desk. I loved that they didn't steer him out but rather welcomed him.

The caregivers sent me a picture of Joe holding the power brick from Reta's electric recliner up to his ear, talking on it like a phone, giving directions to a crew who was working for him. After hearing that, we took his old briefcase to him, filled with papers, a slide ruler, mechanical pencils, gas meter charts, and a pad of paper. When he saw it, he sat right down at a table and got busy, happy to be working again and perhaps even anticipating earning a paycheck. He had seemed worried about money, puzzled by the fact that he had none—this man who had been in the habit of quietly sneaking $20 bills into the pockets or purses of anyone he thought could use a little extra. After watching him search his pockets for a wallet, we found his old one, put in some business cards, his expired driver's license, and a few dollars and took it to him, along with a ring of keys. When Twyla made a personal check out to him for $600 (with "do not cash" on the signature line), Joe tucked it safely into his wallet as well and visibly settled down with these familiar things back in his possession. I saw him lean over and whisper to Reta, "We've got some money. We can go anywhere we want to."

One night shortly after this, Troy took the time to tell Joe that everything was in order. "Joe, we found the file you left for us, and we've followed your instructions. You worked hard and made good plans for the future. There's plenty of money, and all the bills are paid. Everything is taken care of; you did a really good job." Troy seemed to know that he needed to hear these words, and Joe listened carefully, his eyes never leaving Troy's as he spoke. This would be just one of many times that Troy would have this conversation with him. He even at some point let Joe know that we had followed his example and set up a similar file with our own information in it for our kids. We never before understood the real importance of having these things in order, earlier rather than later.

Joe went from working with his briefcase on one day to being back in the army on the next. One caregiver told me about the time that Joe told her, "Soldier! Get to the barracks!" She knew to do what he said, and the closest place was the kitchen, so she ducked in there. He followed her and said, "I *said* get to the barracks!"

She said, "Papaw, I don't know where the barracks are!"

She spent many late nights with him, having midnight snacks and playing with apps on her iPhone. She loved Joe, and he loved her. For a few minutes that one day, he thought she was a soldier, and to us, she was. She was a skilled warrior, serving and protecting not a country, but a man.

Still, Joe loved taking care of people. Around this time, a new resident named Beauna moved in. She was lost and confused, as many were when they first arrived. The girls told me that Joe walked over to her and handed her the baby doll. Reta no longer needed the doll; she was settled now and paid little attention to her. Beauna took the baby, and just like Reta had done a couple of years before, settled right in to taking care of her; she had a job to do.

A couple of days after Christmas, Twyla called me at work to tell me Reta had a seizure. When I got there, she had been cleaned up and was resting in her chair, exhausted from the experience. I really believed she was dying but learned this is a normal process on the Alz journey. Her brain was dying and triggering events. In my mind, I pictured short circuits. She had at least two more seizures at Delano House, each one taking a toll on her.

Joe kept a close eye on Reta to be sure she was receiving proper care. I was in the habit of telling him when I left, "Thank you for taking care of Mom. I love you." In the beginning, Joe would say he loved me too, or he would thank me. This was our routine. One day, when I said goodbye to him, he said, "I need to go see my Mama." Reta was sitting right next to him. I didn't try to correct him on this sort of thing; I just told him I would see him tomorrow. He said, "I'll miss you. I need to go see my Mama."

I wasn't sure if he was talking about Reta or his grandmother who raised him. I told him I would miss him, too, and to travel safely; I gave him a kiss and hug, and left.

14

More Chaos and Confusion

It was hard to believe so much time had passed, and it was already January of 2015. I asked Joe about Sadie, the yellow lab who belonged to one of the caregivers. Sadie visited often and knew Joe would feed her anything she wanted, even tuna sandwiches and nacho cheese Doritos. They were great pals. He thought real hard and asked, "Did I leave her with you?" which made me wonder if he remembered his Chihuahua for a minute. As worried as I was about him leaving his dog behind, he had never asked about her or looked for her, at least not that we recognized. We decided to bring him a stuffed dog, as we had given Reta the baby doll.

Joe didn't only love dogs and cats; he loved all sorts of creatures, even spiders. He picked up a black origami tarantula in the office one day, handling it very tenderly, and petting it as if it were real. One caregiver heard him say to the spider, "Hey, guy, where's your Mama?"

The caregiver said, "Papaw, that's my boyfriend!"

Joe said, "Oh, my gosh," and continued holding the spider and talking to him while listening to boyfriend stories.

The next day, Joe had his stuffed dog in his lap, wrapping it carefully in a warm blanket. He loved this dog and believed it was real. It had a Christmas hat sewn on its head, and it must have been sewn well because Joe never gave up twisting and pulling, trying to get that hat off. One day when I was there, he handed the dog to me and said, "I think he's sick. Can we take him to the doctor?"

I agreed with him. Seemed reasonable, I thought, since the dog wasn't moving, barking, eating, or blinking—could be sick.

On January 5th, we celebrated Reta's birthday. She was happy—a lot of the usual gibberish plus a few distinct words. At the table, she reached for my hand and spent time intertwining our fingers and then lifted our hands to her mouth, kissed my hand, and smiled at me. It was such a tender moment; it had not happened before and didn't happen again. Troy heard her say something about a little girl and thought she knew me that day.

When I was leaving one day in late January, I told Joe I was going home to fix supper and I would see him tomorrow.

He said, "Haven't you been here about a year?"

I paused and said, "Yes, it's been almost a year."

He said, "Well, make it easy on yourself."

I wasn't sure if he understood at that moment where we were, but I found it so interesting that he had the timing right. It had been a year since he had arrived at Delano House.

Things had changed a lot in a year for both Joe and Reta. Reta had a good year, such an improvement since we moved her, largely due, we believed, to the stimulation she was experiencing at Delano House. It was hard to believe. I loved seeing her dressed and sitting at the table for meals, smiling and trying to communicate. The decline was happening, no doubt, but this had been a good year, with some time reclaimed for her. Joe, on the other hand, was declining quickly. It may seem insignificant, but two indicators to me that he was going downhill were when he quit wearing his boots and later when he quit wearing his jeans. Seldom in my life had I seen him in anything other than boots and jeans, but now snaps and zippers were challenging, and boots were a struggle to pull on and off. Things were changing.

Joe seemed more confused at times. I asked him one night, "What did you have for supper?"

He thought about it for a few seconds, and said, "I don't remember."

I asked if he had seen Sadie that day, and his answer was, "I don't remember."

No matter what I asked him, he said he didn't remember and looked as if he was really focusing hard and trying to pull up those memories, as if he knew he *should* remember. When I asked about Reta, he frowned and looked as if he was thinking very hard. He finally said, "I don't know what I'm supposed to be doing. I don't think anything's wrong with me now."

I got his briefcase, opened it up, and looked at some things with him. When he finally shifted his attention more toward that, I left. I sat in my car in the dark parking lot, eyes closed, head against the headrest, for several minutes before driving home.

Thankfully, every day was new with things in a constant state of change, and many times, the change was good! A couple of days after that depressing "I don't remember" visit, Joe was very friendly and talkative. We sat in the living room visiting, with Reta reclining by his side. At some point, Troy signaled to me that he was going to the restroom. When he stood up and turned to go, Joe said, "I guess you don't want to talk about that anymore?"

It was so surprising, so different from my conversation with him a couple of days before. As Troy walked away, Joe said, "That's the best man I ever . . . wall."

Again, when Troy was walking back toward us, Joe said, "He's a good man. The best man I ever . . . jaw."

An ad for Classic Country music came on TV, and we heard Patsy Cline singing "I Fall to Pieces." When Troy asked Joe if he knew who that was, Joe sang along for a bit but couldn't quite come up with the name.

I asked, "Do you think it's Patsy Cline?"

Joe said, "Yes! It's Puppy Kitties!" We all laughed out loud, and it felt good! Reta was awake, enjoying our conversation, smiling and chuckling. At one point, Joe looked at her and motioned for her to come closer and said, "Come over here, Mama." Later he reached over, patted her and said, "You're doing fine, Mama."

He had reached across the couch in Big Lake and said this to her many times.

The men were definitely outnumbered by the women at Delano House, and for a long period of time, Joe was the only man. He had many interesting encounters with the ladies; some made me laugh while others gave me pause. In August, I bought four or five new shirts for Joe's birthday and took them to Delano House for him. Beauna (the one Joe had given the baby doll to) by this time believed Joe was her husband. Poor Joe; he always needed someone to take care of, and he was very good at it. Beauna claimed him as her own, truly believed it, and I think Joe believed it about half the time. Sometimes they held hands. I didn't like it, but I knew Joe would always be loyal to Reta, as much as his brain would allow. When I spread the shirts out on a table to show him, Beauna walked over with him and proceeded to tell me that he didn't like the color on one, the sleeves on another, the logo on another, pointing to each as she delivered her verdict. She was quite serious about it and told me to return them to the store right away. There was a mixture of happiness and confusion in Joe's eyes—happiness over seeing me, especially with new shirts, but confusion over this woman telling me to return the shirts to the store. He looked at me, shrugged a little, and turned to study Beauna for a minute. I could picture him thinking, "This is Reta, right? Or is that Reta over there in the recliner? Why doesn't Reta like my shirts?" I just smiled, agreed with her, and then walked to Joe's room and hung them up in his closet. Everyone was happy.

Before Beauna, there was Irene. She was in very good shape physically, and she and Joe were two of the only ones who could talk and walk around freely when Joe first got there. They became friends and enjoyed one another's company. Before long, I believe Irene either thought he was her husband, or she was willing to just pretend he was, whether Joe knew it or not. I had to remind myself that Joe wasn't thinking clearly and would never hurt Reta. We have a few family pictures with Irene in them, and Reta too of course! She was always happy to see us and believed she was part of our family, and we didn't tell her differently. I told myself that Irene didn't understand that Joe didn't belong to her. Then one day, I watched as the hospice aide, trying to move Reta from the recliner to the wheelchair, called over her shoulder to the other caregivers, "Hey, can someone help me with Reta?" Irene happened to be walking by about that time, and said to her, "I would help you, but that would be . . . *awkward.*" Maybe she wasn't all that confused after all.

At the Thanksgiving potluck meal, Beauna wanted to be close to Joe. A caregiver tried to steer her away from our family and toward her own, but Beauna said, "*You* go visit with them; I'm staying right here!" The caregivers tried everything, but nothing worked. Beauna's family finally ended up coming to our table, and her daughter said, "I guess when you've got it, you've got it!"

The caregivers always said Joe was a chick magnet; I guess he was. He was indeed handsome, had gorgeous blue eyes, and was very friendly.

A few days later when I was there, Beauna walked up behind Joe and put her arms over his shoulders, resting her forearms on his chest, leaning down so that her face brushed his. I was nervous, watching Reta. She was sitting there with us but had her eyes closed, and I hoped she was unaware of what was happening. The caregivers tried several ways to get Beauna away from Joe. They tried the baby doll, which Beauna was very attached to, but she simply said,

"You go feed him." Nothing worked. They told her that I was Joe's daughter and that Reta was his wife.

She said, "OK," and whispered to Joe, "Did you hear what they said?"

Joe smiled. No wonder he was confused.

Even though Irene had declined so much, she still loved Joe too. Seeing Beauna by Joe bothered her some. Later that day, Joe walked by Irene and said to her, "I'm not going to bother you," and kept walking.

Irene said, "I wish you *would* bother me!"

It made me think of high school with one cute guy in a class full of girls, a lucky situation for the guy!

Another very sweet resident there was Lenora, and thankfully she never declared Joe as her own. One day, for some reason, Joe very quietly got up from the dining table, picked up a pitcher of water, walked over to Lenora, and proceeded to slowly pour the water on her head, as if he were watering a plant.

Lenora was such a sweet lady, always smiling. I could imagine her saying, "Thank you," if she had words to speak. One of the girls got up quickly, grabbed the pitcher of water away from Joe, and he chased her down the hall to get it back! I would love to know what he was thinking.

There were times when he fought the girls, usually when they had to take him to the bathroom. They understood this was difficult for him and had learned to duck when he swung. He connected a few times and no doubt it hurt; he was very strong. He wouldn't have purposely hurt them for anything, and once when he realized he had, he couldn't stop saying, "Oh, baby, baby, baby, baby."

Joe didn't see many men at Delano House, and his pre-Alz world was mostly men. One man who came to Delano House faithfully every night to feed his mother and get her ready for bed became a friend to Joe. When Joe saw him walk in, his slight, manly nod toward the door spoke volumes, and as his friend shook Joe's hand and asked how work had been that day, Joe's eyes sparkled, believing this was an old friend who still came to visit him every night.

A true friend from the past, about ten years older than Joe, made the great effort to visit one day. Although Joe couldn't communicate with words that day, he made it clear how happy he was to see his old buddy. It was apparent in his eyes, smile, handshakes, and hugs. Only when I walked him to the door after the visit did his friend shed a tear. It wasn't easy for him to make this visit, and I realized he could teach the rest of us a few things about making time for others.

Joe was a smart man. He knew he was losing the ability to communicate and recognized that the time was coming when he would no longer be able to convey his love and appreciation to me. Eventually, when I said my usual "goodbye" and "thank you for taking care of Mom" as I was leaving, he would use all his energy to hold on to me, look deeply into my eyes to be absolutely sure I listened and *really* heard him, as he said, "I love . . . you . . . with . . . every . . . thing." It was a struggle to get those words out. Our time was getting shorter.

15

Tears and Goodbyes

On Reta's 82nd birthday, I made a fruit cocktail cake for everyone to share. This cake had been served by my grandmother many times; she had made it often, and so had Reta. On this day, however, it was brand new to Reta, but she enjoyed every bite. She relaxed in her recliner that day, with a slight smile on her face, leaning a bit toward the kitchen. She loved hearing the caregivers' conversations as they were preparing meals or washing dishes. These were familiar sounds to her, and she loved them.

It was so strange, with both Joe and Reta, to see them give up on silverware and start eating with their fingers. It seemed with both that there were three stages: feeding independently with utensils, feeding independently without utensils (including some coaching with the first bites), and then being totally dependent on others for being fed. The last stage was long for Reta but fairly short for Joe. The first time I saw him pick up pureed chicken fried steak and gravy with his hands and eat, it was clear that we were well into this Alz journey.

Mealtimes were always interesting. One night, I was sitting beside Joe while he ate supper when one of the residents must have gotten it in her mind that Joe was her late husband, and she was very irritated with him.

"You're eating like a hog!" she said. "Don't you know we don't have the money for that?"

Joe was clueless and just continued eating.

"Stop that! You don't need anything else to eat! I *said* that's *enough!*"

And on and on. I had to laugh; it was an amusing scene to watch, and Joe's oblivion made it extra enjoyable.

Chatting with these folks was easy and fun and brought genuine smiles to their faces. One day, one was smoothing out a quilt on her lap, imagining she was preparing to cut a pattern for a dress. She looked surprised to see me and said, "Mama and I were just talking about you, wondering how you were doing! How are the girls?"

I said, "They're growing like weeds!" It was easier to do this than to try to explain that I wasn't who she thought I was. It simply served no purpose. I remembered Troy's uncle standing in the hall talking to the mirror years earlier and wished I could have another chance to chat with him.

Whether or not she understood it, Reta heard me tell her I was her daughter at least once a week. Sometimes it was obvious she didn't believe me, and other times, she seemed glad to know it. Most of the time, however, it didn't really matter to her one way or the other. It was around the end of March 2016 when I was feeding her a hamburger and fries, and I reminded her again, "Do you know I'm your daughter?"

She responded, "Nope."

"I am. My name is Tracie Marie."

She looked at me, perplexed and maybe a little suspicious. "Hmmm."

I pressed on. "You're a great mom."

With a tiny bit of a smile, she responded, "Good."

That day when we left Delano House, as I was saying goodbye to Joe, I told him, "I love you; you're a good man."

I smiled when he so earnestly responded, "*You're* a good man!"

On April 3, I went to Delano House to spend some time with Reta, but she didn't seem to feel well. She wasn't laughing or smiling or trying to communicate, as she usually did when I fed her lunch. About halfway through the meal, she threw up, not a lot but enough to ruin her food and make it clear to all of us that she didn't feel well. The girls immediately took her from the table, freshened her up, and brought her back shortly with new, clean clothes on and got her settled in the recliner. I sat with her for a while, but she wasn't her usual self; she seemed tired. I eventually left so she could rest and called back later to check on her. She hadn't gotten sick anymore and was resting comfortably. All was well; maybe she was coming down with a virus.

The next morning, when my phone rang at 5 and I saw that it was Twyla calling, I braced myself for bad news, perhaps another seizure. As soon as I answered, I heard Twyla sobbing. She said, "Mama's gone. I'm so sorry! Tracie, Mama's gone."

I couldn't believe what I was hearing. I was just there; I knew she wasn't feeling well, but I didn't expect this. It's strange. We had been on this journey to the end for a long time, but the news still stunned me.

The caregivers cried with me as we sat in her room. She looked so peaceful, confusion and frustration finally gone. It was good to spend some time with her. I talked to her, touched her, hugged her, and really cried. The hospice aide asked if I would mind if she bathed her and put fresh clothes on her before the funeral home arrived, so I stepped out as she began to gently tend to Reta, her touch filled with love and respect.

Troy and Byron came, and we all sat in the stillness of her room, as reality slowly sank in. One of the girls had opened the window in her room, a tradition started years earlier by one of the caregivers so the person's spirit could leave. Eventually, the funeral home came to pick her up, but I stepped out of the room. I had seen her arrive on a stretcher but didn't want to watch her leave on one.

The caregivers did a good job of keeping things as low-key as possible when one of the residents had passed away, but each time, Joe seemed to know. Even though other residents didn't notice, Joe did. Sometimes he stood outside of a resident's room, refusing to leave, standing guard until death came. Thankfully, though, he was unaware this time. He had slept late and never knew the funeral home came to pick up her body. When he did get up, the girls showered him with love and a yummy breakfast. I watched from a distance, not wanting Joe to see my swollen eyes and tear-stained face. He was well cared for and completely unaware of the fact that, this side of Heaven, he wouldn't see his true love again.

Even though I had seen Reta almost every day for the past two and a half years, she hadn't known me for a long time. Still, she was happy to see me, loved having the company, even if I was someone she hadn't met before. Even though she hadn't known *me*, I had known *her*, and I would miss seeing her, touching her, hearing her little chuckle, and even hearing her say she didn't know who I was. I had started missing her years ago, but now I really, truly missed her. I was thankful to know that the body I saw then was only a shell, like a locust leaves his shell behind when he flies away. Mostly, I was thankful for the assurance of meeting her again one day in the home God himself had prepared for us.

I hoped we could just sail through this. Maybe Joe wouldn't notice or remember her. But after a couple of days, Twyla called and said she thought I needed to tell him, that he was looking for Reta. He had been standing in front of her chair, with tears on his face; he couldn't figure out where she was. I was sure, still, that with a few more days, we would be able to move on. I wanted this to go away so I wouldn't have to have this conversation with Joe.

A few days later when I was there, Joe was frustrated and distraught. He was in one of his "trying so hard to figure things out" moods, really frowning, thinking so hard, and he said several things I didn't understand. Once he said, "I don't know what to say." Then he said, "I can't figure it out." And he looked at me, eyes pleading, like he was thinking, "Please help me figure this out!"

I wished Troy were with me, but I knew I had to move forward with this conversation by myself. "Dad, are you missing Mom?"

He said emphatically, "Yes, I am."

I said, "Dad, Mom passed away; she's in Heaven now. It's just us; we'll stick together and take care of each other; we'll see Mom again when we get to Heaven. You live close to Troy and me. And we will all take care of each other now." I had pictured myself strong, comforting him, but I wasn't. As my tears fell, he reached for me and pulled my head down to his chest and rubbed my back, saying, "It's OK. We're going to be OK."

I wasn't comforting my Dad; he was my Daddy again for a few minutes, and he was comforting *me*. It seemed like my tears would have dried up by then, but they kept spilling over, soaking Joe's shirt.

The caregivers told me that one day, shortly after my visit with him, Joe stopped in the kitchen and looked at Reta's picture on the fridge, removed the magnets that held it in place, and held it in his hands. They cried when he started singing George Jones's song "He Stopped Loving Her Today." So many words were locked away in his mind, like prisoners under lock and key, but these escaped easily that day—making it clear that, through it all, he still loved her and hoped she would come back to him again.

16

In Time for a Dance

When we walked in, Joe saw us from a distance, and as soon as I saw his eyes, I knew we were going to have a problem. I had told Troy that since Reta had passed away, I thought Joe saw her when he looked at me. He had started calling me "Mama." It seemed strange because there were so many days when he didn't seem to know who she was, sitting right next to him. I wonder now if a younger version of his Reta was easier for him to identify.

There was joy in his eyes as they locked on mine. I mean pure joy, and by the time I got to him, tears were dripping from his face to his shirt. He grasped my arms and murmured, shaking his head slowly. "I can't believe it," he said. "You're here. I can't believe you're here with me. I can't believe it."

There was no doubt that he thought I was Reta; the tears wouldn't stop. When he couldn't seem to focus on anything else, I moved behind him and began giving him a shoulder rub. Troy sat in front of him and talked to him, trying to steer his mind to different thoughts. Joe was distracted though, looking around the room for me, or rather "Mama." He asked Troy where I went, worried and pressing Troy for information. "Am I going crazy? Where is she? Where did she go?"

Gently, Troy told him, holding his hands, "Joe, I think you thought Tracie was Reta. She looks a lot like her." A couple of minutes passed before I moved in front of him, but he didn't notice me; his eyes were still searching the room.

Joe seemed to lose ground more quickly after Reta was gone. Not only did he miss her, but I wondered, after so many years of attentive caregiving, if he had lost his purpose for living. He had loved her unconditionally, and she had lived well and safely because of him.

Eventually, however, it was time for him to get back to work. When the maintenance man came to work on the dishwasher, Joe was his assistant. He got down on the floor, looking under the sink, and worked along with him. At one point along the way, Twyla sent me a picture of Joe on the floor, on his back, under a wheelchair "working" on it, as he had done with so many cars in his life. One of the caregivers bought him a child's set of tools in a tool box, and this kept him busy for quite a while. In his mind, there were many projects that needed to be worked on, and it was good for him to be needed.

Joe had played the guitar in his younger days. He was quite talented and even played for a short period of time at Lubbock's famous Cotton Club in the company of some well-known country and western musicians. We kept his guitar at Delano House, and he loved getting it out occasionally to play a little. One night, there was someone there singing and playing for a resident's birthday, so I got the guitar out so Joe could join in. His strong fingers, still scarred from a fire long ago, easily found their familiar places on the old strings, but then just froze there, unable to move. He looked up at me like a frightened child, realizing he didn't know what to do next. There was sorrow in his eyes as he handed the beloved, well-worn instrument to me. We both understood that his fingers would never again find their places on those old strings.

He had always loved music and often sang around the house. In the fall of 2016, we bought some cheap, wireless headphones for him and connected them to classic country music and country gospel.

It seemed to stir something in his brain as he sang and spoke a few words clearly; it was an amazing experience. We ended up buying a second set so there would always be a pair charged and ready. Joe sang along often, and we loved hearing his voice and seeing a new twinkle in his eyes.

He began walking constantly; he could not make himself stop. He was losing some of the strength in his legs, and it made everyone nervous to see him walking, no longer sure-footed. He sometimes stopped suddenly and leaned way back, far enough back that it looked like he would just topple over backward like a stack of blocks. The more he walked, the wearier he got. The caregivers tried to coax him to sit down, but if he sat, it was only for seconds; then he was up and going again.

One day, Twyla called me at work and said they couldn't get him to stop and were afraid he would fall and hurt himself. When I got there, they had just gotten him to sit in a rocker, but he was frustrated and tired, yearning to walk. Twyla sat beside him, worried, tears streaming down her face. I got on my knees in front of him and started rocking the chair with my hands, essentially trapping him in the chair. When he leaned to get up, I just acted like he was leaning up to give me a hug. I hugged him and kept rocking as he leaned back again with a heavy sigh. I sang to him, talked to him, rocking and hugging. Finally, after two hours, he drifted off to sleep, and I went back to work. I heard later that his nap was just a catnap; he was up and going again within minutes after I left.

Over a period of just a few weeks, Joe went from this constant walking to not being able to walk at all. He lost all strength in his legs and was, for the most part, in a wheelchair. It was strange how quickly this happened. Watching the girls move him from the recliner to the wheelchair was bizarre to me: he had no ability to command his legs. I remembered the time Troy and I had tried to move Reta, but her feet seemed glued to the floor. It was like watching a rerun of an old TV show that I really didn't want to see again. I wanted to turn the channel. Joe loved moving around, and it was heartbreaking to see him trapped in a body that wouldn't allow him to do what he wanted.

It was late August, close to bedtime, when Joe had his first seizure. When one of the caregivers spotted him from across the room, she ran and lay on top of him to calm him down and keep him from hurting himself. The girls told me that as soon as the seizure was over, he said "Mama." He was delirious with high fever, and he moaned deeply in his sleep. I took the next day off and sat in his room with him all day, playing music, singing, talking to him, and resting. I believed he was dying, and I think the girls did too. A couple of them who no longer worked there came by to see him, and I knew they had been called. After about 24 hours, he woke up and was ready to get up.

The seizure had taken a toll on him, and he began choking when he ate and many times when he drank. His swallow reflexes weren't working right; his brain was losing track of this function.

A few short days later, Joe fell and hit his head. When Troy and I took him to get stitches, he acted like a little kid in the car, excitedly pushing all the buttons on the dash the whole way, as if he had never seen so many buttons before. It was a very deep gash, just above his left eyebrow, requiring eight stitches, but Joe was strong, never giving any indication that it hurt. I felt like a mother, worried over my boy lying under the hands of the doctor as she stitched him up, as if she were repairing the seam in an old shirt. It was soon after this that we started hospice care.

In early November, Twyla called me at work. Joe was having another seizure. I left work and spent the afternoon there with him. The nurse explained that his heartbeat was getting very erratic, and his oxygen level was low, which meant that his brain was getting less and less oxygen. She explained that this is part of the process with the brain dying. She was surprised he hadn't had more seizures and said she expected more to come. He was still very strong physically, but definitely losing ground quickly.

Delano House had a family meal in mid-November to celebrate Thanksgiving. It was a potluck meal, the kind they did regularly for celebrating holidays with family. I made Reta's apple cake, which was one of Joe's favorites. He wasn't very aware of us being there and certainly wasn't aware of the apple cake. He sat at the table with us, and we took turns feeding him.

Joe's decline over the next two weeks was significant. His pain was increasing. He couldn't communicate details, but from his body language we knew that he was hurting more and more. His pain meds had been gradually increased but weren't keeping up. The hospice nurse told me that most people on the amount of medicine he was getting would be literally knocked out. I gave permission for more frequent morphine, and not just as a last resort. Once they were able to determine an appropriate level, morphine became his normal scheduled medication. It absorbed quickly and provided fast relief, but each dose only lasted three hours. I knew it would make him lethargic but felt that we had stretched this out as long as we could; I couldn't bear to see him hurt much more.

He was in a lot of pain one day as they were still monitoring and adjusting med levels. Pain was clear to us mainly by his labored breathing and furrowed brow. Even so, he talked the entire time and was trying to communicate something to Troy. Troy couldn't understand him but took the time again to look him in the eye and tell him clearly that everything was OK, that everything was taken care of, that he had done a good job. We weren't sure how much Joe understood, but he really looked at Troy and seemed to be listening. Usually, when Joe talked and we had no idea what he was saying, we just answered him, one way or another: "That sounds good, Dad," or "We'll have to look into that." On this day, Joe was talking so much and so focused on Troy, that Troy finally had to say, "I sure wish I knew what you were saying!"

Joe said, "Somethin', somethin', somethin'," and he and Troy both chuckled.

On Christmas Eve, I took Joe outside in the wheelchair and played Christmas music. The weather was gorgeous; we didn't talk much, just enjoyed the peace and quiet, the cool, crisp air, and listened to the Christmas story through the words of "Silent Night" and "Hark! The Herald Angels Sing." I shared some things with him that day that were weighing on my heart. He wasn't able to offer any advice, but he listened. He was still my dad, still the one I could go to, and I felt better after talking to him. He was calm and happy, just the two of us. It will be a good memory forever.

His next seizure was in the recliner a couple of days later. The girls called and told me I should come. They first thought he had passed away in the chair, but when they jostled him, shook him, talked to him, and moved him out of the chair, his eyes opened. His response was minimal, however, so they moved him to his bed and called hospice.

He was unable to swallow, and we knew his time was short. Hospice came and explained everything to us, saying it could be a couple of days, or it could be a month. I knew I couldn't bear it if he lived for a month, unable to eat or drink, and prayed for God to take him home and end his suffering. We were with him around the clock from that point forward and arranged for two of the caregivers to stay with him overnight so we could sleep as well. We didn't know how long it would go on, knew we had to stay rested and healthy, but didn't want Joe to open his eyes and see an empty room. I was actually on his bed, straightening his covers, trying to make him more comfortable when he said to me clearly, "Thank you, hon." Still, he was showing his love and appreciation to me—I loved him so much.

Troy spent the first night with Joe even though a caregiver was on duty that night. She walked into the room, and told Troy, "I'm kind of embarrassed to do this with you here, but this is our usual thing. I like to do this with Papaw." She climbed on his bed, lay beside him, and started singing to him, along with the country gospel music we were playing. Troy said it was very moving, hearing her sing the words to an old favorite from the past, "I'll Fly Away." As she sang the familiar words about a place where joy never ends, Troy knew her soothing voice brought him comfort and perhaps even hope that there truly would be just a few more weary days.

Around December 31, our son Brad came over to see Joe. I believe Joe heard Brad when he prayed, and it was a sweet, emotional time. I will never forget Brad's tender, heartfelt words about the impact he knew Joe had on Reta's life and how all of our lives (mine, my children's, and my grandchildren's) were different because of his true love for Reta.

On January 3rd, it had been six days since Joe had lost his ability to swallow. We had been swabbing his mouth with a wet sponge, but he wasn't able to eat anything. When we first started this, his lips locked around the sponge as he sucked every drop of water from it. Gradually, the desperate clamping down on the sponge weakened to simply an open mouth as we pressed the sponge against the inside of his cheeks, forcing the water out. During these six days, he had no food and only about three ounces of water.

Troy pulled a chair up close to Joe's bed, took one of his hands, and leaned down close to him. "Joe, I want to explain something to you. I know you, and I know that you would want me to tell you this. You're not able to swallow anymore, and this is the reason you aren't able to have food and only very little water. Your body is starting to shut down, Joe, and soon, you'll be able to join Reta in Heaven."

We believed he could hear Troy's words, but we weren't sure.

Troy continued, "We love you, Joe. You're a good man. Every-thing here is taken care of. It's OK for you to go to Reta; she will be so happy to see you. Her birthday is in two days. Wouldn't it be great to make it in time for a birthday dance?"

I knew it was hard for Troy to do this, but he knew Joe's ana-lytical mind would want to know what was happening. Hearing these words from someone he trusted, I believe, brought comfort to him. He didn't have to fear the unknown; now he knew he was preparing to leave his physical body behind and would soon join his sweetheart in Heaven. It reminded me of years earlier when Joe was honest and open with Reta, talking about her disease, while holding her hand and telling her, "It's going to be OK, Mama."

I stayed with Joe, talked to him, hugged him, held his hand, sang to him, and kissed him. That afternoon, Twyla suggested that I go home for a little bit and rest. She said that Joe might need me to leave, that often fathers just won't pass away with daughters in the room. I wasn't sure about this but did understand that he might want some space. I kissed his forehead, told him I loved him, and that I would be back in a bit.

I had been home for about an hour when Twyla texted me and said I should come on back. Within five minutes, I was on my way out the door when they called and said, "You should come now. I don't think it will be long."

When I walked in, the girls met me at the door, tears spill-ing from their eyes, reaching to embrace me. He was gone. Twyla believed that he heard them call me, understood that I was on my way, and did not want me to be there to see him pass away. I wasn't sure how I felt about us having that kind of control, but it did sound like a decision he would make if that were possible. My heart ached deeply and I missed him instantly. I touched him, kissed him, smoothed his hair into place, straightened his collar, and cried, remembering his last words to me: "Thank you, hon." He was finally at peace; the battle was over, the giant slain. The caregivers grieved too; we all loved him.

The girls said Joe was a real man, and Joe and Reta's love was a real love. They had witnessed this true love which had raised the bar for what they looked for in a man. One told her husband, "I want a love like Mamaw and Papaw." Another told me, "It was so touching to see the love in their eyes for one another. I'll never forget his feet propped up on her recliner or his reaching over to tuck her blanket under her shoulders. Sometimes, we would catch Reta smiling, just looking around in case he was nearby. When she responded to nothing else, she came to life, warmed up by the sound of Papaw's voice. I truly want a love like theirs. Everybody should be able to experience that."

What an amazing man he was, caring for his bride as she faced Alzheimer's, even as he felt himself beginning to lose the same battle. I love him for taking such sweet and tender care of her. I like to picture her waiting at the door to Heaven, as she had waited at Delano House for him, smiling and reaching for him as he walked in, only this time, each recognizing the other, with new and perfect minds and bodies. Their earthly journey was complete, and it was time for a birthday dance.

A time to weep, and a time to laugh, a time
to mourn and a time to dance.
—Ecclesiastes 3:4

Afterword

Looking back, although the journey was hard and I would rather have skipped it, I know others have had more difficult roads to travel, whether with Alzheimer's, cancer, heart disease, or even situations that have nothing to do with illness, but rather heartache. Everyone's experience is different. I have met people whose care for their aging parents doesn't look anything like my story. I recognize that this book might have been written differently, or maybe not at all, if not for the kind of people Joe and Reta were. I'm thankful.

I've thought many times over the years about how we all anticipate parts of life. For instance, we think about and plan for graduating from high school, attending and graduating from college, getting married, having children, even retiring and having grandchildren. But, I realized, no one talks about reaching the part of life when our parents need our help and what exactly that means. I truly did not give it much thought until the time was here, and then I began to stumble through the process, figuring it out as I went, as I believe many others do.

The last half of 2014 and most of 2015 were especially difficult, and I was exhausted, physically and emotionally. When I went to the doctor for my yearly check-up, she asked how things were going, and I burst into tears. I guess there was more stress than I realized. I went through a bit of depression, I think, but that is part of the real story for most people who travel this unpredictable road with people they love.

Although it was hard, I wouldn't trade those last three years, in particular, for anything. There were long periods of time when neither of them knew us, but their eyes lit up when they saw us walk in. They knew that, whoever we were, we were there to see them, and it made them happy. I am thankful for so much time spent with them, even for the times when no words were spoken, but hands were held.

Thankfully, mixed in with the heartache and stress, there were many moments of joy, like the births of six grandchildren, reminding me that there was life outside of the Alz world I was living in. I had much to be thankful for. Each baby brought a breath of fresh air and new energy, not only to us but also to Joe and Reta. Even if they didn't know their names, these babies brought smiles to their faces, joy to their hearts. I love the memory of Joe looking at six-month-old Eleanor and saying, "She's got a full thing of cuteness!"

I made mistakes along the way; there are some things I would do differently had I known then what I know now. I learned a few practical things, nothing others haven't also figured out. Some worked only for a short period but made a difference when we needed it. Some that worked for me may not work for others, but there's no reason for each of us to struggle alone, trying to figure it out. I remember feeling comforted when friends shared their own stories with me, like I had others walking beside me on this journey. I hope that by sharing my own story and the words below, you also feel comforted, that you find something that makes a difference, and reminds you that you are not the only one traveling this road. To learn more about me, my story, the book, Alzheimer's disease support, our family, our faith, and more, visit my blog at https://traciebevers.com.

* * *

I heard someone describe our memories as layers of sand, with the deepest layer being our earliest memories. Our more recent memories are layered on top, in the order of occurrence, with the last meal or last conversation, for instance, being the top layer. Alzheimer's is constantly sweeping layers, beginning with the top ones or the most recent memories, so they aren't there for long. Soon, the only memories left are those deeper layers, from long ago. This explained why Joe and Reta both kept insisting they needed to go home; they were remembering childhood homes, a deep layer that was now a top layer. Neither, at some point, believed the house they were in was their home. I thought of these words many times along the way, and they were helpful to me.

Websites, Books, and Articles

Shortly after I shared my Alz journey with coworkers, a friend sent me the book *Still Alice* by Lisa Genova. I cannot recommend it highly enough. It changed everything for me. I was finally able to let go of trying to pull memories back to the surface. I finally understood those memories were simply gone. Reading this book took a lot of pressure off both me and my parents.

Another book I read soon after Reta's diagnosis was *The 36-Hour Day* by Nancy L. Mace. This is an excellent resource, a practical guide for caring for someone with dementia.

Keeping Love Alive as Memories Fade by Gary Chapman is a book I recently ran across that has excellent reviews. It's on my list to read soon.

There is a wealth of information on the Alzheimer's Association website (www.alz.org); I highly recommend spending time there. This is where I first went to learn more and found the stages of the disease and figured out where we were on our journey. Dig deep, and you will find much, including warning signs and symptoms, stages of the disease, caregiver support, treatments, risk factors, clinical trial information, and more. Check your local chapter via this site to connect with a support group.

When you go to the Alzheimer's Association site, you will find a link to the Walk to End Alz. I recommend getting involved. Helping raise money for the Alzheimer's cause may be a worthwhile way to spend some of your time. Whether or not you raise funds, I found that connecting with so many others on the same journey was a healing experience.

Grain Brain by Dr. David Perlmutter is an interesting read that will make you think more about how nutrition affects our brain health.

Dr. Dominic D'Agostino is a neuroscience, molecular pharmacology, and physiology researcher. He is very interesting to listen to on the topic of how our brain is impacted by what we eat. Look for his YouTube videos.

Teepa Snow (www.teepasnow.com) is a fantastic speaker and teacher with a passion for teaching others about dementia. Look for her YouTube videos as well. I didn't learn about her until late in our journey.

Genetic testing is discussed in many circles. It is something each person must decide on his own; educate yourself so you can make a wise decision. This document mentions the possible impact on employment, health insurance, and long-term care insurance; I had not thought of those factors before reading the article. (https://www.alz.org/documents_custom/statements/genetic_testing.pdf)

There are many ways to love your brain and reduce your risk of Alzheimer's disease and other dementias. These should be easy things for most of us to do, and we should be motivated if we have family members with Alz. I have to continually remind myself of the importance of diet and exercise. (https://www.alz.org/brain-health/10_ways-to-love-your-brain.asp)

Behaviors may vary greatly between morning and evening, and recognizing this and planning around it when possible will make a difference for all, patient and caregiver alike. This is called sundowning. One out of five people with Alzheimer's disease will experience Sundown Syndrome. (http://www.webmd.com/alzheimers/guide/manage-sundowning#1)

Medicare, Home Health Care, and Hospice

There's so much to know about Medicare and health insurance. It's not easy to figure out and certainly not an easy task for those facing dementia. It's important to learn what you can. These websites are a good starting point:

http://www.alz.org/care/alzheimers-dementia-medicare.asp
www.medicare.gov

Home health care may be a great option for many healthcare services that can be offered in the home. It usually is not considered a long-term solution but is helpful to many for a period of time. It certainly was for us. (https://www.medicare.gov/what-medicare-covers/home-health-care/home-health-care-what-is-it-what-to-expect.html)

Hospice care is a form of medical care that focuses on comfort and quality of life for the patient facing a terminal illness. Reta's time on hospice was long, over two years, but Joe's was only a couple of months. They supported not only my parents, but the rest of our family as well. (https://www.verywell.com/what-is-hospice-care-1132618)

Financial and Legal Matters

There's much to know about financial matters, and no one's situation is the same. Some types of care are not covered by Medicare and can create a financial burden for families. Following is a website that may be helpful as you trudge through information and search for options: http://www.alz.org/care/alzheimers-dementia-costs-paying-for-care.asp.

If your loved one is a veteran, or the spouse of a veteran, you may qualify for assistance with healthcare and/or burial benefits through the VA. Search for a VA Advocate in your area for assistance with the application process. Don't try to do it on your own; most advocates do not charge for their services. (https://www.va.gov/)

The Social Security Representative Payee program provides a system for managing Social Security payments for your loved ones who are incapable of doing so. You will be required to do an annual report, but it is very simple. (https://www.ssa.gov/payee/)

Locate the following legal documents while your loved one can assist you: birth certificate, marriage certificate, divorce papers, insurance policies (including long-term care, health, and life), banking information (including CDs, bonds, stocks, etc.), discharge papers from the service, retirement plans, annuities, deeds and titles to property and vehicles, tax returns, safe deposit boxes, log-in and password information to online accounts, etc. Here are some websites to help you:

http://www.alz.org/care/alzheimers-dementia-planning-ahead.asp
http://www.alz.org/care/alzheimers-dementia-legal-documents.asp
http://departingdecisions.com/beforedeath-checklist/

For documents that are not in place, Legal Zoom is a good resource for simple documents, but must be done early in the process. There's much to learn! I did not know that the Power-of-Attorney document I used for many purposes, including paying bills, was null and void after Joe's death. I ran into a snag or two with one bank because I could no longer use this document, and I was not listed as a beneficiary on his bank account. (https://www.legalzoom.com)

Remember: this may also be a good time for you to put these documents together for yourself so that you are prepared for this conversation with your family in the future. We were surprised to find that Joe had prepared most of these documents ahead of time for us, and we followed his example and did the same.

Death

A friend recommended that we contact Ken Lambert via www
.funeralnegotiator.com.

We used this process, and it worked very well for us. Don't
wait until death occurs. It will relieve much stress and will also save
you money if this is taken care of well ahead of time. They do the
groundwork to find the best option for what you are looking for
in a funeral, regardless of the location. It was a relief, when death
came, that these details had all been handled, and that we had been
wise stewards of their money.

It's hard to believe we have to think about fraud prevention too,
but identity thieves actually target people who have passed away. Be
sure to contact credit bureaus after death to be sure your loved one's
identity is protected. (http://www.creditcards.com/credit-card-news
/how-to-prevent-id-theft-after-death-1282.php)

You may also find this checklist helpful: https://www.verywell
.com/survivors-checklist-after-death-1132601

Little Things

It took me a while to get comfortable with such mayhem in conversations. I finally learned that it was OK to have no idea what
to say at times or how to respond when Reta asked me a question
that I didn't understand. I learned that it was most important to
just be there, hold her hand, tell her that she was beautiful, and
just talk about anything—from the weather to flowers to birthday
cakes. With Joe, I found myself saying often, "That sounds good,"
or "I'm not sure; I'll have to check on that." And he was satisfied;
I didn't have to know exactly what he had said. There were times
when just sitting quietly was perfect; I sat beside Joe many times
while he was deep in thought. Other times, if the silence was awkward, I just talked to them about what happened that day, what the
kids were doing, or work, whether or not they responded. If they

laughed, I laughed. I didn't have to know what was funny. Even with other folks, I learned that it was OK if one thought I was her granddaughter. What difference did it really make?

When we figured out that we weren't getting mail because the post office couldn't read Reta's writing, I printed up sheets of address labels with our address on them so she could just stick them on envelopes to mail to us. I printed return address labels for her too. I didn't know at the time that Alz was the reason for the change in her handwriting, but regardless, this was a good tool for a period of time.

When we started hearing more and more about missed appointments and so forth, we bought a large calendar for the wall (like 20"x30") and started writing everything down, from birthdays to appointments. We did this for several years, and Joe really depended on it.

At some point along the way, Troy and I each put a business card in Joe's wallet, each with notes on them: "Joe's daughter—call in case of emergency," that sort of thing. They were never used, but they were there in case he was in an accident or got lost and couldn't give the information needed. Looking back, maybe there were even times it was helpful to Joe to look at them and be reminded of who we were.

We took family photos and put them on the fridge, in magnetic plastic sleeves, with our names on them. This was Troy's idea, a way for them to look and be reminded of family members, what they looked like, what their names were. A Shutterfly book of family pictures is another great idea. (www.shutterfly.com)

Check to see if your area has Meals on Wheels. It is a fantastic program that delivers hot meals to those in need. When Reta was well, she delivered many meals to the folks in her town, but I was never able to convince Joe to receive them when they were needed.

Shortly after Reta's diagnosis, for her birthday I made a scrapbook filled with pictures, mostly of her parents and brothers and other family members, young pictures of her, some of me as a baby, along with handwritten recipes from her mother. She loved looking at it, would lean over each page, closely studying and touching each picture. This became something we could talk to her about. We took it with us for every visit for a while, and each time, she seemed to think she was seeing it for the first time. The day nothing about it registered with her or interested her was sad, but we had used it for a long time; it's a precious keepsake for me now.

One of my ideas that was a mistake had to do with an old rolodex of phone numbers and addresses. Joe and Reta had used this rolodex for years, along with other contact info written on the inside of the phone book, and still other info written on sticky notes in various places around the house. I decided to organize all that information in a binder. It was well done, typed, organized alphabetically, each sheet in a plastic sleeve and easy to use. Unfortunately, Reta could never quit looking for the sticky notes or notes written in the phone book. This was probably the first time it became clear to me that it was important for things to be the same, unchanged, consistent. I regretted doing it but couldn't un-do it.

When Reta began wandering from the house, I ordered a Safe Return bracelet for her. As it turned out, she went into the nursing home about the time we received it, so she never wore it. It's an excellent idea, and I highly recommend it. We should have ordered it sooner. Search for it on the www.alz.org site.

On our quest for a system that worked for keeping Joe on track with medicine, one thing we tried was a Pill Organizer with Alarm Reminder. It is a great tool and can work, depending on the circumstances. Joe really hated it after a few days, and I was surprised it didn't end up in the trash. But I still think it can be a good solution for many. I found it on Amazon.

Doll Therapy, Other Activities, and Sensory Toys

This is a great article about the use of baby dolls for both men and women with dementia. Joe, by the way, loved the baby as much as Reta did. (This baby still lives at Delano House!) We did not purchase an expensive doll, but just a lifelike baby doll at Walmart for less than $20. This site has other great information about activities for Alz patients including puzzles, games, and sensory toys. (http://www.best-alzheimers-products.com/category/alternative -therapy-for-alzheimers/doll-therapy-for-alzheimers-disease)

You may also find great options at educational toy stores (such as the Lakeshore Learning Store), things made for children but perfect for dementia patients. Some of these items are Dressing Frames, Lacing Cards, Giant Beads and Laces, other sensory/activity boards, and so on. Someone made a board for Joe with various locks and latches on it. Be sure items are not small enough to fit in mouths. (That may seem obvious, but it wasn't to me until the day I had to take Reta's wedding band home because she was putting it in her mouth.) Check out www.lakeshorelearning.com.

There are some good ideas here—many are homemade. (https:// www.pinterest.com/explore/alzheimers-activities/)

Also, remember simple things like a briefcase, wallet, keys, maybe a baseball to hold. Large Lego blocks and puzzles with large pieces work well, as do coloring books.

Remember music! The wireless headphones were a great experience for Joe, and I wish we had tried them earlier in the process. We bought ours on Amazon, and they were cheap—about $20. I suggest that you search YouTube videos that show the difference music makes with these patients. There is a difference, by the way, between listening to music being played in a room vs. listening on the headphones, where all other sounds are blocked. It is amazing!

A friend recommended Rachael Hale's picture books to have on hand for Joe and Reta to look at. Both loved them and spent many hours during their illness studying these pictures of babies and animals. The pictures are also great conversation starters.

I'll Love You Forever by Robert Munsch is a children's book that has nothing to do with Alzheimer's but everything to do with love and caregiving. It was a favorite of my kids when they were little, so I gave each of them a copy after Reta passed away. We were living the story.

* * *

Most Important of All

The Bible is the best resource by far, and I found myself going there time and again. You might also find that reading the Bible aloud to your loved one not only stirs memories from years past but soothes fear and brings hope. The words are powerful, true, and unchanging—far different from the doubt, suspicion, and mayhem that have taken up residence in the minds of our loved ones.

You are my hiding place, you will protect me from trouble and surround me with songs of deliverance.
—Psalm 32:7

Giving Thanks

Thank you to Troy, who not only took good care of Mom and Dad, but also took special care of me along the way. Hearts were stirred when others witnessed your love for Mom and Dad, the strength they drew from having you near them, hearing your voice. You have truly set the bar high for others on this long road to goodbye. I'll love you always.

Thank you to Brad, Jessica, Byron, Kacie, and Deidre for walking beside me on this journey, for recognizing how precious and short time is, for understanding time focused on Mom and Dad, and for listening to me and sharing many tears. *"I'll love you forever, I'll like you for always."**

Thank you to all of our extended family, including my precious mother-in-law, Ann, who never failed to encourage me and to pray for me.

Thank you to Therese, who made a real difference in this journey, first by sharing *Still Alice* with me and second by leading us to the place that became home for Mom and Dad.

Thank you to Twyla and her team. . .the ones I eventually started calling "lovegivers" instead of "caregivers." You became the hands and feet of the perfect protector, safekeeper, and love giver to Mom and

* Robert Munsch, *Love You Forever* (Willowdale, ON: Firefly Books, 2001).

Dad. You provided a home for them when they reached the point of needing help keeping each other "in sickness and in health." Your love is sincere and felt by all who enter your home.

Thank you to the folks in Big Lake who loved Mom and Dad, watched over them, and protected them. . .even as Dad managed to hide the truth from us. Because of you, they were able to stay in their beloved Big Lake well beyond what would have been possible otherwise.

Thank you to many, many friends who listened to my stories, shared tears, gave warm hugs, and said prayers.

Thank you to Laura Allnutt and Lucid Books for challenging me to dig deep and for helping me discover a love for writing.

Mostly, I give thanks to God. The long and rocky road to good-bye was hard, but I knew it was not too hard for Him and that He walked the road with me. . .carried me, mostly.

Ah, Lord God! It is you who have made the heavens
and the earth by your great power and by your outstretched arm!
Nothing is too hard for you.
—Jeremiah 32:17 (ESV)

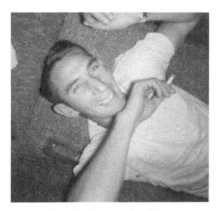

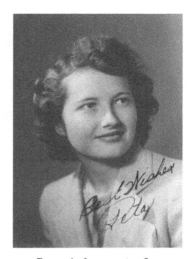

Joe – before meeting Reta   Reta – before meeting Joe

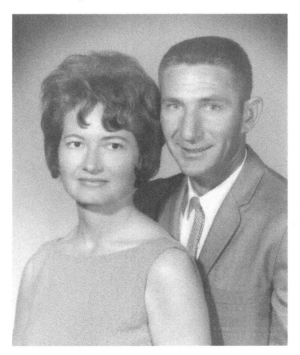

Newlyweds in 1964

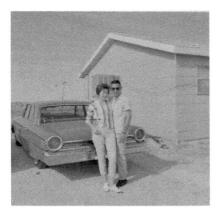

The 60's, Proud owners of a red Falcon

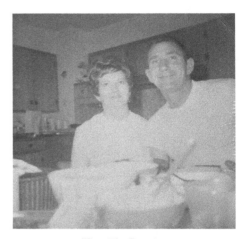

The 60's, Pure joy

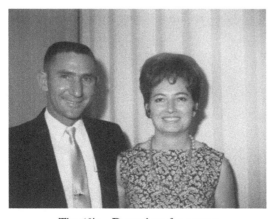

The 60's – Dressed up for a party

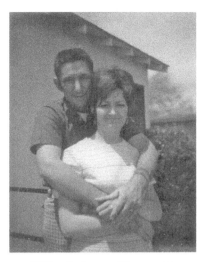

1973 – Both were 39 years old

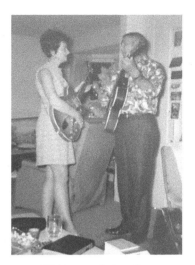

Making music together

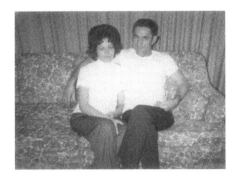

The 70's, Midland

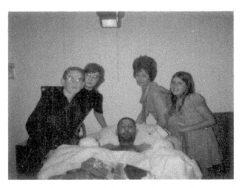

Celebrating Christmas after the fire

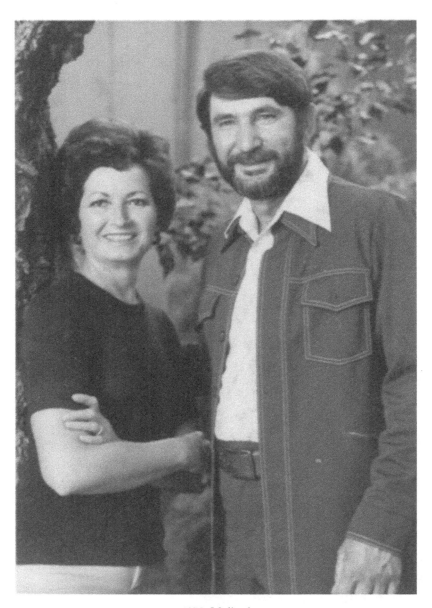

1978, Midland

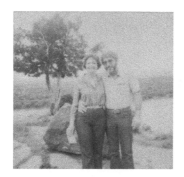

The 80's, Lake Buchanan

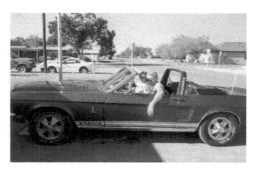

The 90's – Riding in the Shelby

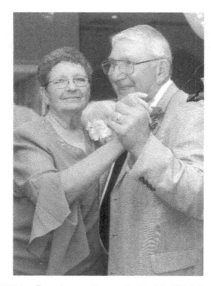

2006 – Dancing at Byron & Kacie's Wedding

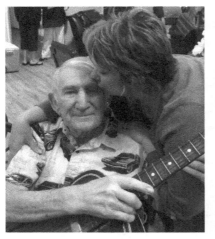

Still loving the guitar

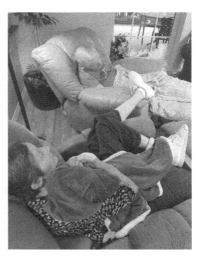

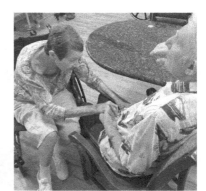

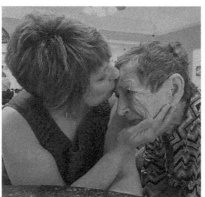

Did you know you're my Mama?

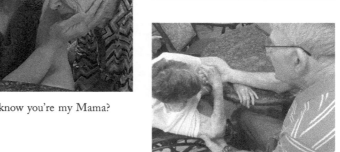

Sweethearts, together again

Has this world been so kind to you that you should leave with regret?
There are better things ahead than any we leave behind.

—C.S. Lewis

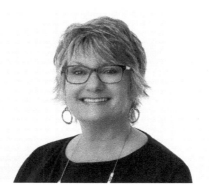

Tracie Bevers spent well over a decade journeying through the world of Alzheimer's after her parents were diagnosed. She learned a lot about real, true love and treasuring time, which is precious and short. Along the way, she became passionate about sharing information with others just beginning their own journey to goodbye. She has known her best friend, Troy, since she was 14 years old and has been happily married to him for many years. They have six grandchildren, and she loves making new memories with her family and storing them away for the future, a love that grew stronger after her experience with her parents.

CPSIA information can be obtained
at www.ICGtesting.com
Printed in the USA
FFHW011048271018
48960980-53200FF